AF824232

Counterfeit Cure

M. Roman Slavin

Rockwood Press • Philadelphia, PA
2013

Rockwood Press
Philadelphia, PA
Copyright © 2013 by M. Roman Slavin

All rights reserved. No part of this book may be used, reproduced in any manner whatsoever, stored in a retrieval system, or transmitted, in any form or by any means, electronic, mechanical, photocopying, recording, or otherwise, without prior written permission from the author.

ISBN: 978-0-9888786-1-7

Dedication

For Cliff, love of my life and consummate professional.

An estimated 30-50 percent of the global medicine supply chain is counterfeit. (Source: World Health Organization)

"... nearly 40 percent of the drugs Americans take are imported and nearly 80 percent of the active ingredients in the drugs on the American market come from overseas sources." (Source: remarks given by Margaret A. Hamburg M.D., FDA Commissioner in October 2010)

Drug counterfeiting is a $35 billion-per-year business. (Source: World Health Organization)

A person convicted of distributing counterfeit drugs can expect a jail sentence of approximately 2 years. (Source: FDA)

That same person convicted of distributing illegal drugs can expect a jail sentence of approximately 10 years. (Source: Drugwarfacts.org)

Although FDA field inspections have increased, the Agency's budget is in danger of being slashed due to U.S. austerity measures imposed by politicians.

Chapter 1

Before Kat finished reading the latest MedWatch reports, the ailing, the suffering and the limp baby bodies were seared into her brain, there when she closed her eyes, there when she stared at the screen in disbelief. These were the kind of cases that brought back bad memories, twisted up her judgment and exactly the kind of cases she joined the FDA to work. She tried hard to shake off the images, square her brain, maybe get some sleep since the last thing Dan needed in a lead FDA investigator was flawed judgment. The stories haunted her until she finally gave up and got ready to hit the road, anxious to start digging for mountains of good, hard evidence. She shivered. Those mountains were going to be high.

Thanks to Bernie, the last ten crawling miles of traffic were the exasperating result of leaving late, in spite of her best efforts at an early start. He didn't care that she had timed the trip perfectly to avoid the Maryland/D.C. traffic and get to Philadelphia before the evening rush. All he cared about was that he was out in the yard and he wasn't going to get in the Explorer until he was good and ready. Kat had learned that lesson only minutes after adopting him three years ago but she still held out hope that one day she would triumph over a 62-pound coonhound more interested in sniffing out all the wildlife in the neighborhood than obeying commands.

"How you doin' Bernie?" Kat asked as she spied him in the rear view mirror.

Bernie snorted, opened one eye and closed it again.

He was sacked out of the back deck of the truck, lulled to sleep by what was now the constant hum of the engine as the traffic cleared. Kat sailed the rest of the way through Delaware. Good thing Dan approved back-to-back meetings with Blank and TemePhelps in Philadelphia; it gave her an excuse to spend some time with Albe while she was in town.

She had planned to drop Bernie off at the kennel, but as soon as Albe found out, he insisted that she bring along his furry little brother and let him stay at the frat house with him and the rest of his buddies. What could be better than hanging out with a bunch of rowdy, smelly, frat boys? Kat glanced back Bernie. For as much as he annoyed her, the thought of anything happening to him made her grit her teeth to stop tears from welling up.

Two years after Jorge's death, Albe started in on her about a companion to keep her company when he was off at college. Kat knew he meant a new husband, but she chose to believe that he was encouraging her to get a pet. Finally, she searched the kennel for a nice cat and in the process, walked past Bernie's cage and was smitten. That hound so obviously flirted with her that even the attendant commented. He flashed his big golden brown eyes and hung his head so his floppy ears almost touched the floor and let out a pathetic whimper that stopped her in her tracks. She left the shelter with him, or more accurately, being dragged out by him. Afterwards she learned that hounds were some of the toughest dogs to train, and coonhounds... well, forget it. They're loud, boisterous, smelly hunting machines, who also happen to love to drape themselves over you if you sit still for more than ten minutes. Kat learned to adjust her expectations of how a dog should behave. Why not? She just spent the last five years adjusting her life expectations after the Jorge's murder.

She glanced back at Bernie one more time. That barking, mess of a crazy dog still was the cutest thing when he was asleep, and he was a great distraction. As Kat settled back into the drive, her mind wandered back to the reports.

They had started piling up only recently, a rash of incidents presenting as allergic reactions along with a stack of suspected substandard efficacies, all centered in her region. Usually investigations turned up a bad lot, a contaminant, or real world results only discovered after pre-market testing. Pretty predictable stuff. But something about this cluster of cases got under her skin, and ever since Jorge, Kat had learned to listen to her gut.

She forced her attention to the music on her iPod, just as Patsy Cline belted out a tune and skipped forward until she found Lyle Lovett singing about Texas and settled into the rest of her drive. When her thoughts drifted back to her open cases they inevitably led to Jorge and the greedy fuck who murdered him. These new cases smacked of Klein or some shit like him. She still woke up some nights in a cold sweat, sobbing, repenting for not being a better pharmacist, for not knowing that something was wrong with his meds, and mostly for not protecting him. How could she have missed the signs? How could she *not* have known that his pain meds were shorted?

"Mr. Klein, is it your testimony that you diluted out the prescribed doses of medication because you couldn't make a profit if you had filled them properly?"

"Yes."

"Explain this to the court."

"First of all, if you look at the oncology literature, you will see that the drug is still effective at the lower concentration. And, using the lower concentration allowed me to still make money. The government's guidelines for reimbursement haven't kept up with the cost of drug and the cost to me for filling the drug. So, what, I'm supposed to supply this for free or for negative money? Talk to your Senator if you want the health care system straightened out. I'm just one guy. I didn't do anything wrong."

Every time Kat thought back to that arrogant snake in the courtroom, she couldn't help but wish that his life in prison was a miserable nightmare at best. It wasn't just that he was a colleague who acted in such blatant violation of the pharmacy oath and all that was right and decent, but that he wasn't even sorry for it. The other victims and their survivors seemed to heal better, but Kat wasn't cut out for forgiveness, not when she knew exactly the pressures Klein was under and the profession he chose.

"Listen honey," said Sheila Klein as she approached Kat after the verdict, "you just don't understand how hard it was for my Joel…"

Kat stopped listening to the woman, jammed her hands into her pockets to keep from wrapping them around Sheila Klein's neck and waited until her mouth stopped moving. Then she lit in to her.

"You, with your fake fingernails, your botoxed face, your fur coat, Louis Vuitton bags, Mercedes and whatever else you worship above human life, are on your way to the wrath of God. You got that?"

She still remembered the blank look on the woman's face and how she regretted wasting her breath. Dan Smithson was only an FDA investigator back then, but he happened to be in court that day and couldn't help but overhear.

"You're a pharmacist, right?" he had asked her after introducing himself.

"Mmhmm."

"I could use someone with your passion on my team."

"I don't think—"

"Don't make any decisions right now. Take some time, and then call me."

He handed her his card and left the courtroom. She tucked the card into her purse and tried to forget it, but every time she thought about Jorge, she thought about Klein, which made her think about Dan. It only took a couple for weeks for her to call. By then, Dan had been promoted to Director of Investigations and was looking to beef up the department. One lunch meeting later, Kat had applied for a job.

She heard what sounded like a steaming teakettle and looked in the rear view mirror to see Bernie standing in the back of the truck, wagging his tail and whining.

"Okay, buddy. Mom's stopping."

Either he had to relieve himself, or he was just bored and wanted to stretch his legs. Either way, she could use the break herself, so she pulled into the next rest stop, climbed out of the truck and walked back to free the hound from his cushy prison in the back of the Explorer. Bernie took off immediately for the overflowing trashcans in the parking lot and gobbled up a half-eaten Roy Rogers burger before she could yank him away. Well, at least he'd be set for food for the next few hours. Then it occurred to her that she should let him forage through the trash some more and get a real bellyful before the frat boys treated him to a bowl of their cheap beer. She would dutifully advise the boys that the dog should not be given beer, and then no doubt find out a few days after she got home that Bernie had spent most of his time in the frat mildly drunk. In the time it took her to consider this thought, Bernie annihilated a hot dog, some fries, two servings of chicken bones, a biscuit, the remainder of a Coke, a candy bar wrapper and a used tissue. She figured that was enough nutrition for one stop and dragged him over to the grassy area to relieve himself, then back to the truck. She coaxed him inside and locked him safely in so she could dash inside for her own quick bathroom break.

"I'll be right back," she said, trying to reassure him, knowing full well it was wasted effort.

She could hear him baying his displeasure all the way to the front doors of the rest stop. Once inside, Kat used the facilities and stared at herself in the mirror while she washed her hands. During her time with Jorge, she was well kept: updated hairstyle, reasonably nice clothes, make-up most of the time, and only a few extra pounds. Since his death, she'd forgotten how to care and now what stared back at her in the mirror was a wrinkled, stretched out Gap T-shirt hiding a frame with an extra twenty pounds, a face beginning to look like her mother's, gray roots and an outgrown bob that hung off her head like a mop. Kat sighed and considered treating herself to a haircut and a day at a spa in Philly.

She picked up a paper, a few snacks and a drink for herself, and then headed back out to the truck. At some point in her absence, Bernie had calmed down enough to change from his bellowing howl to a loud whimper, but as soon as he spotted her coming back, he started up again, startling the guy standing next to her truck. The guy seemed annoyed rather than amused and Kat was about to get up in his face, but remembered Dr. Bunson's anger management techniques and proceeded to get into the truck and drive off without so much as a peep.

After another few minutes on the road, her phone piped up and she struggled to keep control of the truck while she answered it. She quickly considered whether Delaware was a "hands free" state and told Maryann to hang on for a minute while she switched to her earpiece.

"Got it. Now, what's up?" she asked.

"Another case reported that seems like the ones you're already working on. I uploaded it to the database, so you can grab a copy once you get settled," Maryann replied.

Kat sighed heavily and tried to push away the seared images.

"Same class of drug or same drug altogether?" she asked.

"You got, what, so far?" Maryann probed.

"Antibiotics and an anticoagulant," Kat replied, hoping the list wasn't going to get any longer.

"This one looks to be antiarrhythmic," Maryann replied.

"Jesus, what are these guys trying to do, kill everybody?" she shouted as she thumped the steering wheel with the heel of her hand.

"No casualties that we know of. Just reports of allergic reactions and reduced efficacy," Maryann said.

"Got that on the antibiotic too, but I haven't ruled out resistant strains of bacteria yet," Kat said.

"Where are you on the lot testing?"

Kat glanced over at the day planner open on the passenger seat next to her. She had multiple red circles around the dates where the testing began.

"Two weeks in. I should know something in another week or so, but in the meantime, I thought I'd have a little chat with the boys at the manufacturers and see if I pick up any hints from them."

"Oh, and Dan says bring back some Tastykakes," Maryann replied. "Krimpets and Peanut Butter Kandy Kakes."

"You're kidding me, right? Jesus, he's had two heart attacks already. I ought to call his poor wife and let her know," Kat sniffed.

"The Tastykakes are nothing compared to the stress of these MedWatch reports."

That snapped Kat back to reality. She hung up and tried to stop her head from spinning. She gripped the steering wheel until her breathing returned to normal. The cases drifted back into her head before she could brush them aside. With her almost photographic memory, she conjured up case after case, trying the make all the pieces add up.

"Brrrrraaaaawwwwwwccccck!"

Bernie. She laughed out loud at his ridiculous snoring.

"Well, at least one of us can sleep," she muttered.

His minor distraction didn't last long and Kat was back to rolling cases around in her head.

Antibiotics Case One, New Jersey. Physician reported that several of his patients suffered adverse reactions in response to a normal course of the antibiotic, Amoxicillin. Patients experienced skin rashes, dizziness, light-headedness and other allergic type responses not previously noted in studies from TemePhelps, the manufacturer. FDA traced to the pharmacies that filled the scripts, all were notified of immediate quarantine of the remainder of the supply and to prepare for an inspection. TemePhelps was notified of the case and other similar reported cases and informed that the FDA required quarantine of remaining supply, lot testing sample reports, and a pending inspection.

Antibiotics Case Two, Delaware Cases Three through Eight in Pennsylvania and Five through Seven in New Jersey—all the reports were similar, if not identical to the first New Jersey report. All traced back to TemePhelps.

The anticoagulant cases were in sixteen states and growing, mainly centered on complaints of efficacy—there had also been eight fatalities. A number of emergency room physicians and EMTs reported the need to use additional doses of Heparin to achieve the same therapeutic effect. But the data was inconsistent and the efficacy issue did not present in all cases of Heparin during the same time period, though the drug was from the same lot.

Kat checked the clock and hit Brad Wright's cell number on the speed dial.

"I figured you'd be out on the boat," she said, startled that he answered the phone.

"Today's golf day," he replied. .

"So, retirement agrees with you?" It was a rhetorical question. Brad never sounded better. "Got time for some quick questions, for old time's sake?"

"Anything for you, hot shot," he answered.

Kat smiled. Brad was the legendary "Lion" of the department and the standard by which all others were judged. Kat was flattered that he took her under his wing early on, taught her the ropes and hooked her up with some of his sources—, basically, building her reputation. She wasn't sure why, but she was grateful to be his heir apparent and like everyone else, she had been sorry to see him retire last year.

"Any of other guys get in deep when Cantor did?"

"No. Why? What are you on to?" he asked.

"Tracking down a rash of reports right now. Broad range. Just trying to get a handle on them all," she replied. It was clear from his tone that his curiosity was piqued.

"Cantor again?" he asked.

"Not sure yet. Wait! Hang on." A sudden surge of cars surrounded Kat and though she was speeding along at 70 miles per hour, they made her feel like she was standing still. She gripped both hands on the wheel, held to her lane and waited until they all passed before resuming the conversation.

"Sorry, Brad. Goon squad on I-95," she said.

"Ahhh. I don't miss that," he replied.

"So, was Cantor alone? I thought I remembered a number of issues," she asked.

"They were the only one with pharma problems at the time. The others were dog food, lead in toys, and sundry items like toothpaste. Oh, and later it was the baby formula," he replied.

Kat was silent for a moment, pushing the images of limp baby bodies and dead pets out of her head.

"TemePhelps's got Heparin problems now, but it looks like a bad lot to me. I'm not suspecting anything like Cantor, nothing 'back door,'" she said.

"Kat," he said slowly. "Cantor was no accident."

Her fingers clutched the steering wheel. She had known there were suspicions of deliberate tampering but the FDA had no legal reach beyond American borders. She tried not to sound too alarmed.

"Deliberately added?"

"Seemed like they were duped by the Chinese too," he replied. "Drug was being produced in China, real mom and pop. Literally. Couldn't meet demand. Their western educated sons figured out they could use ground up animal cartilage and chemically alter it to show up like heparin in the testing and pass it off. Cantor added it to batches of the drug's active ingredient."

Kat struggled to control her breathing. "You shut anybody down?"

"You're joking, right?" he laughed.

Kat shook her head and rolled her eyes. "Let me guess, Congressional hearings, lots of headlines and no new authority," she said, trying even harder to control her tone.

"That's why you're the hot shot," he said.

"Yeah, if I can figure out how to get Congress to overhaul our budget and grant us the authority we need to get things done right," she said.

"Good luck with that. Call me anytime. And Kat—be careful. You may be playing with some big boys here." His last words were hard to ignore. If Brad was worried, she had better be worried too. Problem was there wasn't too much she could do to make the worry go away. Everyone at the FDA knew they needed additional funding to hire more investigators and more authority to shut down overseas plants. Everyone knew they had to live with only the ability to block the importation of what might be considered "at risk" goods. As soon as one supplier was shut down, the very next shipment of goods was relabeled to look like a different supplier, when in fact it was the same supplier with new paperwork. It killed her to think that anyone would completely disregard the safety of thousands of people in the pursuit of profit, and she was by far the most vocal of the investigators to Dan, to Congress, to the press, and basically to anyone who would stand still long enough to listen.

Now she had some kind of confirmation that these new cases were bigger than some simple mom-and-pop pharmacy case. Far bigger. Brad realized it and so did Dan, but it was up to her to get this solved and fast. Kat ran over the strategy in her head: systematically investigate each likely scenario to conclusion. But, if the reports continued to pile up, she also needed to pursue them concurrently. Likely causes at first brush were falsified or underreported data from the initial testing, a contaminated lot, contaminated or substandard raw material, improper storage issues or just plain negligence. That was just on the manufacturer's side of things. At the pharmacy, the medication could be incorrectly filled, a storage contamination issue, or tampering by some crazy person. Last of all, and probably the least likely, was the possibility of hanky-panky by the manufacturer, sloppiness, or worse still, that the pharmacy was knowingly buying counterfeit drugs. Kat was exhausted, though thinking about the work ahead quickly energized her.

She finally pulled off I-95 on the West Philadelphia exit and made her way to Albe's frat house, a venerable old Victorian in a tree-lined neighborhood near the University of Pennsylvania. What was probably once the summer homes of wealthy Philadelphian's had now become a shabby frat row. Traffic had been surprisingly light, in spite of the impending rush hour; she made better time than anticipated. She hoped that Albe was back from class, so she would have time for a quick visit, to drop off Bernie and get back to the hotel for a long, hot shower. Parking was scarce on the street, but she managed to wedge the Explorer into a spot across from Albe's frat house and unload Bernie from the back. As soon as he got out, he took an enormous dump in the middle of the sidewalk, and then sat next to it, beaming with pride. She burst out laughing, then rummaged through the bags and cases in the back seat of the truck until she found a plastic bag to clean it up. She and Bernie crossed the street to climb the expansive front porch steps of Alpha Sigma Phi house and knocked on the front door. Not surprisingly, the music playing inside the frat house was so loud that no one heard her knock, so she stepped away from the door and called Albe on her cell.

"How much longer?" he asked.

"Bernie and I are on the porch."

He appeared at the door almost before she could hang up the phone and immediately spotted Bernie's "gift." hanging from his mother's hand.

"Aww, you shouldn't have," he said.

Bernie strained at the leash to get to his boy, almost pulling her over, Kat let go and Bernie attacked his human brother with affection. Albe hugged Bernie and submitted to his slobbering, then imitated the whinebarkhowl for which Bernie had become famous in the Vasquez household and throughout the neighborhood. Unfortunately, imitating Bernie's noises only spurred him on and pretty soon the decibel level was louder than the music that poured out of the frat house. It attracted a gathering of fellow frat brothers who piled up at the door to witness the spectacle.

"Bernie's back!" one of them called and the boys whooped and hollered their approval, to which Bernie responded to by ramping up even louder.

Finally, Albe and the frat brothers backed away from the door and let Kat and Bernie enter. She was pleasantly surprised to see that the place was not utter chaos like her last visit, but was actually kind of put together. At least the boys, or probably their girlfriends, had fitted the filthy couches with new slipcovers and a few new side chairs that seemed to have all of their legs intact. Brightly colored fabric covered the walls where beer signs and posters of naked girls once hung and the normal size television had been replaced with one about the side of a small compact car. In front of the set, neatly arranged on a series of tables, were gaming consoles and controllers and a metal rack about five feet tall jammed with the collection of games. A large white board next to the mammoth television announced the scores for any number of electronic contests currently underway. Albe's name was listed only once, a comforting sight. At least he spent some time going to class and doing homework.

"That a gift for us?" one of the new boys asked.

"Ah, a present from Bernie," she replied.

"Here Mom, I'll take care of it," Albe said as he grabbed the bag; Bernie followed close behind.

"So, I like what you've done with the place," Kat said.

"Yeah, one of the many reasons it's been great having Albe living here this year," answered Roger, who reminded Kat of the Otter character Tim Matheson played in Animal House.

"Really? This was his doing?"

She watched as all the frat boys surrounding her nodded in agreement.

"What was my doing?" Albe asked as he and Bernie came back.

"Roger says you're behind the beautification of Alpha Sigma Phi house," answered Kat.

"Well yeah, with some help from Martha."

"Martha as in everyone's Martha, or Martha as in only your Martha?" Kat probed.

She knew Albe hated it when she asked for details about the girls he was seeing and he made his usual face at her. She was undeterred. After all, one of the privileges of parenthood was asking about the girlfriend. There were three other guys in the room: Roger, the new kid, and Jason, Albe's roommate from freshman year. Kat looked at each of them for signs of Albe's seriousness about this Martha. Roger's eyebrows were raised, the new kid just looked stupid, and Jason had a smile that betrayed Albe's secret. Kat looked at Albe and knew immediately that Martha meant something in his life and she felt a little twinge—of what, she just wouldn't admit.

She felt old and little scared, but another thought crossed her mind, one she shook off. She was struck at how much he had grown and how much of a man he had now become. She only had this one child, but she had watched her nieces grow up and it seemed as though the girls were more fully grown in high school before they took off to college. But the boys still looked like boys when they graduated from high school. The change into manhood became noticeable when they returned after their first or second year of college. Now she noticed the change in Albe. His beard was thicker, fuller, his shoulders broader, and the soft layer of baby fat smoothed into more refined muscles of manhood. He even smelled different—not the pungent, ripe smell of young boyhood, but a vague musty smell mingled with the spice, citrus, or woodsy scent of his cologne. It made her think of Jorge in his younger days and it made her clutch a bit.

"You'll meet her," Albe said, cutting off further discussion.

Kat knew from experience that pushing Albe too hard for details only alienated him. Besides, she wanted to drop the subject for her own sake. It had been so hard to let go of Albe and she had to stop herself from running up to Philadelphia every other week to check up on him. Suddenly, her small house had seemed enormous, even with the excessively loud and boisterous Bernie.

"I thought we'd meet up later if that's okay with you. Martha has a late class and then we can grab something to eat after that," he said.

"Sure. Okay. So, I'm going to the hotel, the Holiday Inn on—"

"Mom, I know. I live here, remember?" he finished.

Kat smiled and stifled the impulse to lecture him.

"So, I'll get going. Good to see you again Roger and Jason, and nice to meet you…" she said, sticking out her hand to shake.

"Oh, it's Todd," said the new boy as he stuck out his hand to shake hers.

"Please don't give Bernie any beer, okay? I'm willing to tolerate a lot of things, but that's just not good for the dog and—"

"Got it Mom. No beer for the dog," Albe interjected.

She bit her lip. Sometimes it was just hard to turn off her mother role.

"Okay, so see you later, Bernie," she said as she bent down to hide her face and gave him a kiss on the head. He grunted in what might have been acknowledgement.

"I'll call you later and let you know where to meet us," said Albe.

Kat reached out and got Albe in a tight hug, having missed one when she arrived. To her surprise, he hugged her back, instead of just tolerating her affection. She wasn't sure whether it was because he was growing older or getting kind of serious with a girl named Martha. She had to turn her head quickly so he wouldn't see her face.

***

Jackie DeAngelo escorted a long-haired Russian out of the room and waited for Reggie to thoroughly pat down the next man in line, a small, round, elderly Middle Easterner, before motioning him toward Colton Barnes. The old man was an odd sight in this procession of angry young men, a parade of devilish characters who lined up outside the door, every color, every nationality, every religious affiliation lined up and begging for the same reward. In an instant, Reggie flung the man onto the tile floor and crushed his windpipe with his foot while Gus and Stewart pointed guns at his temple and groin.

"What's the bulge?!" Reggie demanded.

The man struggled to speak under the pressure of the foot. Reggie slowly let up enough for the man to catch his breath and emit some sounds.

"What the fuck you sayin'?" barked Reggie.

The man squirmed and groaned, trying to make himself understood.

"I think he's talking about jewels," suggested Gus.

"Jewels? Is that what you're saying? Jeeewwweeells?" Reggie demanded.

The man nodded and motioned toward his front pocket. Reggie, still with his foot on the man's throat, jammed his hand into the man's pocket and yanked out a black velvet drawstring bag.

"Check for detonators. These fucks like the explosive stuff," offered Stewart.

Keeping a keen eye on him, Reggie felt around the bag and, satisfied, gingerly opened it and pulled out a necklace of deep red garnet stones, each encased in gold filigree; a teardrop pearl about the size of a cashew hung from the center front of the piece. The man made some more noises and pointed to the bag, so Reggie reached in again and pulled out a set of matching dangling earrings.

"My mother, my mother," the man repeated in broken English.

"Must have swiped them from his mother," Reggie said to Colton.

"Either that or sold his mother for them," added Jackie with a laugh.

Colton had been watching the entire event, pretending to be disinterested. He saw that Reggie and the others had the situation under control, but his nerves still remembered the early days, days before the line of men considered him a friend, days when he had to pay attention to everything. Now he sat forward, intrigued at the idea that this man had brought him a lovely gift. He cautiously tamped down the warmhearted feeling that threatened to wash over him.

"Let me see," Colton said as he reached his open hand to Reggie.

Gus and Stewart each stuck a foot on the man and kept their guns poised while Reggie stood up and crossed the room. Colton received the jewelry from Reggie, ran his fingers over the stones, then held the necklace up so the sun could shine through the gems and bounce off the expertly tooled gold. The pieces were exquisite, and he could see that the pure gold and stones the color of blood were crafted by a skilled artisan. Colton envisioned the necklace around Cherie's neck, glimmering against her freshly tanned skin, highlighting her pitch-black hair that fell just below her shoulders and pointed downward to her plump, perfect breasts. He stashed the necklace back inside the velvet sack. Next, he surveyed the earrings and concluded that the same skilled craftsman could not have made them. More importantly, Cherie would not like how the heavy stones would pull on her delicate ears. He thought for a moment about giving them to his mother, but was struck with her sharp tongue as quickly as he thought of her—*'Did you buy that or steal some retarded kid's craft project?"* He winced. No, he would keep the necklace and return the earrings. The man would leave with tales of the generosity and thoughtfulness of The Money Man.

He motioned to Gus and Stewart to let the man rise and approach. They yanked him to his feet and steered him in Colton's direction. Before he could make it too close to Colton, Reggie grabbed him by the arm and stopped him.

"Far enough," he growled.

The man, disheveled from his rendezvous with the floor, complied with Reggie's order and stood two yards away from Colton. He hastily straightened himself up and bowed. Colton dipped his head slightly in response.

"Nice of you to bring me a gift," said Colton.

"You are very welcome," the man replied.

"So, say."

"The Palestinian people, my people, deserve a homeland. We will fight…"

Colton tried never to care about the causes, or the men who dumped them at his feet, ever since his beloved Badia. Even now he struggled to find the words to describe her beauty. Raven hair, full lips, almond-shaped gray green eyes that tunneled deep into his soul. He had never felt so deeply about a woman and, for the first time ever, he had hesitated to approach her. It was the first time he felt beads of sweat on his upper lip just at the sight of her. She came with a gaggle of friends, invited, no doubt, by star receiver Letroy Benson. It was years ago but the hurt of losing her still felt like it happened just moments before. Colton delivered the "refreshments" to the party—coke, weed, some pills, and a bottle of Scotch for himself. He hadn't planned on staying for long but after spotting the beauty, he revised his schedule.

"…our fight will never be over…" the man continued, bring Colton back to the present.

He regarded the Palestinian and tried to focus on his words. The man groveled at his feet, begging, and Colton relished the respect. After losing his Badia, his reason for being The Money Man, was this, now, the worship from the aggrieved of the world. Buoyed, he would carry those feelings home with him, conjure them up, and use them to make up for his bad memories, for his disappointed father.

Since early this morning, he had freely dispensed excess USA Distributors profits to those who came begging. He tried to ignore that they were used for guns, bombs, bribes, whores, and mayhem. He justified his feigned ignorance because, like a junkie, he craved the feeling from these sessions. Word got out quickly that he insisted on being seen and spoken to—the recipient of their passionate requests in person. They must convince him that he should support their cause with his donation. They must make him understand how much his support means to them. They must show that they understood who he was. Even in the underground, there were rules.

He could tell when it was time for another trip to St. Bart's, not just from the USA Distributors balance sheet, but also from the way he felt out of sorts. Maybe there was too much time with Langford or Jackie or a bad night with Cherie. He could never exactly tell. It would start with the daydreams, stabbing thoughts from the University of Pennsylvania days, and progress into twisted dreams and finally no sleep at all. He needed his parade in St. Bart's, craved the attention, the respect, the feeling that he was not inferior to Langford Wentworth or Jackie DeAngelo. Besides, Langford was effeminate and Jackie was now fat. He sucked in his gut and flexed his biceps. At least he tried to still keep in shape.

Colton turned his attention back to the parade in front of him. Though it was good foreplay, he was growing weary and drifted off as the man spoke, focusing on the necklace in his lap and the vision of Cherie wearing it and nothing else.

"Fifty," Colton declared suddenly, interrupting the man.

"You sure," questioned Hugh McNaughton as he peered over the top of his glasses.

"You questioning me?" he shot.

"Of course not, but—" Hugh fumbled.

"But nothing. I said fifty. The man brought me a gift," Colton insisted.

Before he could even turn his attention back to the Palestinian, the man spoke.

"You will be remembered always, you are a man of greatness—"

"These were your mother's jewels?" Colton interrupted, holding up the necklace.

"My mother *made* them," the man said proudly.

Colton ran his fingers over them.

"Ohhh, she made them. She some kind of jeweler or something?" he asked.

"Artist. The gold, it is Jewish and Christian," the man said, and then smiled. "From synagogues and churches," he added.

Colton put the necklace back down in his lap, sat forward and asked, "You stole the gold?"

The man nodded. Colton sat back and smirked.

"Gold cup or gold plate, gold things… whatever they have… then we melt it down," the man continued.

"But taken, stolen, from churches and synagogues?" Colton said tapping on the necklace in his lap.

"Yes, yes. We are poor men. How else do we get gold?" the man said.

Colton threw his head back and laughed. Reggie and the others tightened and the room waited in silence until he explained himself.

"It's like, *sacred* gold or something. My private sacred gold." Colton enjoyed this thought of sacred gold for Cherie. He gripped the necklace hard, imagining the pained faces of worshippers without their gold. "I might make it a hundred!" he suddenly blurted out.

"Ah, now—" Hugh began.

"Don't worry. I know fifty's the top," Colton said to Hugh, then turned back to the man and continued, "Fifty to you old man."

Though seven 30-foot yachts brought down boxes of cash from ports in Boston, Philadelphia, and Baltimore for him to distribute, there was still a limit to how much he could dole out to any single sniveler.

The Palestinian bowed and approached Colton. Reggie jumped forward, stopping him with a firm grip on both his arms. The Palestinian spoke rapidly in his language, words of gratitude, or perhaps a curse, Colton would never know.

"Please, I will approach?" he asked.

Colton gave a tiny nod to Reggie who loosened his grasp of the man. The man dropped to his knees, crawled forward and began to kiss Colton's feet.

"Your sons and their sons will know the gratitude of our people," he murmured in English.

Colton motioned for Reggie to lead the man away, then pointed to a large cardboard box labeled Scott Toilet Paper. Reggie tore open one side, pulled out three packages of bills, closed up the box and backed away, motioning to the man to take the box with him. The Palestinian groaned and grunted as he struggled to lift it. Reggie motioned for Gus and Stewart to help, but the three together still could not move the money-laden box. Finally, Reggie stepped in, yanked the side of the box and managed to drag it a few inches. Gus, Stewart, and the Palestinian pushed from behind while Reggie continued to pull.

In the middle of the rumpus, Colton focused on Hugh, who had been sitting in the corner, computer on his lap, recording the day's proceedings on The Money Man spreadsheet. Hugh heaved a sigh, adjusted his glasses, then entered the fifty into the spreadsheet. The screen flashed as the total of today's offerings recalculated.

"One hundred more left, right HM?"

Colton loved to amaze Hugh at how he kept a running tally of the money in his head. A mind for details was part of his genius. At the end of the day, he always knew exactly how much more could be distributed.

"Mmmmmm," Hugh answered nodding.

Colton smiled. The only way to control his men was to make sure they understood how much he paid attention, even when it seemed that he didn't.

Finally, the Palestinian and his box of money were pushed out of the room and Jackie brought in the next one in line. He was a small, Asian man with a cocky walk and a sneer on his face. He entered the room as though he belonged there and Colton didn't like the look of him.

"State your case," Jackie barked.

"Give me money," the guy said.

Colton narrowed his eyes and slid upright in his chair.

"Repeat that?" he asked.

"I saaaiiidddd, give… me… monnnneeey," he reiterated.

With just a tiny movement of his head, Colton signaled that this arrogant beggar was not worthy. Reggie rushed over, grabbed the man's arms and pulled them tight behind his back. The man did not resist, instead he sneered and laughed. Then Reggie flung him face down on the floor.

"Who the fuck are you?!" Colton demanded.

"So, I'm badass like the rest of these punks and I'm lookin' for some ah, funding," the man answered with a snicker.

Colton bolted from his seat and kicked the man hard in the face, knocking out two of his teeth. The man collapsed into a heap on the floor, blood gushing from his mouth and pooling around him.

"You think this is a joke! You think this is funny? I'm your one big chance to get money for whatever shitbag group you hang with. If they sent you here, they know how important I am. You go back to them empty handed and see how long you live!"

Colton's rubber soles squeaked on the tile floor as he paced around the room, around the man bleeding on the floor, walking off his anger. Suddenly, he charged at the man and kicked him in the ribs.

"Get him out of here," he hissed to Reggie.

Reggie, with Gus's help, dragged the man out of the room, throwing him into the hallway in front of the line of men waiting. He landed with a thud and a groan. Reggie slammed the door and helped Gus wipe up the blood.

Colton stood in front of the window and looked out at the ocean, willing his anger away, trying to regulate his heavy breathing. He could leave now, he should leave now, but then he would have to finish this business tomorrow and one day of this was enough. Jackie tapped him on the elbow and offered a bottle of whiskey. Colton brushed it away with the back of his hand. Jackie continued to stand next to him at the window, still holding the bottle. Colton concentrated on the soothing ocean view in front of him, focused on the lapping waves and the sprinkling of boats close to the shore. A couple of minutes passed, his breathing returned to normal and finally he accepted the bottle and took a long swig. The burn felt good going down his gullet, he closed his eyes and savored it. Calmer now, he returned to his seat and motioned for the next one in line.

Jackie ushered in a very tall, very black man wearing some kind of traditional African garb and positioned him in front of Colton.

"Colton, this is Kunle—"

"No names, Jackie!"

"Sorry. Sorry. Uh, this is your next appointment."

It irritated Colton that Jackie could do his job well, but often didn't. Colton kept him around in spite of his shortcomings, because Jackie was much smarter than he and always was. But now, it was Colton who ran Jackie. For all the years he had known him, Colton had always thought of Jackie as a good friend. There were a few times he felt genuine affection for Jackie, but somehow he was always disappointed. He could forgive the screw-ups, but not the humiliations. As the humiliations piled up, he considered Jackie more of a useful acquaintance than a friend.

"Thanks to your previous generosity, we have been successful in our crusade, but this time now is critical. We are needing more weapons…"

Colton's mind wandered away from this very black man with a very thick accent from Somalia or wherever who stood before him, to the view out the window where topless women strode along the milky white sands while the crystal blue ocean lapped at their perfectly manicured feet. For the first time he regarded the women out there with idle attention because Cherie was with him, because he was thinking of marrying Cherie. He turned back to considering what seemed to be an endless line outside his door and pressed his eyes shut. All he wanted to think of now was Cherie and how glad he was that he had brought her. It was risky exposing her to his other life but if she were marriage material, he had to know that she could be the kind of wife he needed. Her reaction to his St. Bart's world would be a deal breaker.

Right now, the thought of her lounging near his pool, clad in nothing but a bikini, made him impatient. It was time for the parade to end.

"Tally?" Colton asked Hugh.

"One hundred left," Hugh replied.

"Jackie, what's the count out there?"

Jackie strained to look out the window at the remaining line.

"Ah, eight more," he reported.

"Twenty packs," Colton said to Hugh who dutifully recorded the transaction on his spreadsheet, then motioned for Reggie to hand the Somali the appropriate number of bundles. Reggie reached inside a cardboard box and counted out twenty bundles, then handed them to the Somali, who came equipped with his own inconspicuous straw beach bag and colorful beach towel to drape over the top of the open bag. Each pack of bills totaled $10,000 in a variety of denominations, to make it easier to be quickly spent. Colton always liked dirty bills, always loved the moldy, musky smell of used money.

"Move it along, Jackie."

Jackie waddled across the room behind the Somali, opened the door and called for the next one in line. Colton snickered and remember back when Jackie and his father came to him begging for help after Jackie's father had racked up a mountain of gambling debts and managed to piss off his bookies enough to earn a contract on his head. Jackie Sr. wanted Colton to ask his father, Daddy Joe Barnes, for the money, like he was some kind of errand boy. He probably thought that a former pro football coach had extra cash just lying around waiting for some sucker to come asking. Colton had curled his hands into fists as they spoke. Jackie Jr. knew full well that Colton never brought messages to his father and never spoke him about business or money.

Colton eyed up Jackie Sr., was about to explode from listening to his pitch, when it occurred to him that he could legitimize the money from his street drug business by bailing Jackie Sr. out, and in the process, grab a controlling interest in USA Distributors. Overnight, Colton had gone from street drug dealer to owner of one of the largest legitimate wholesale drug distributorships on the east coast, and member of the rich and famous crowd himself. Jackie, once the heir apparent to his father's business, was now relegated to being Colton's right-hand man. His growing gut showed how much it bothered him to be second in command. Like his father, he swallowed his troubles along with his pasta, sauces, meats, bitter greens, crusty breads, and rich desserts.

Jackie tried to fight every new way Colton ran the business, said he couldn't stomach the thought that they were lacing the legitimate drug supply with counterfeits, but he never objected to the money. In fact, when Colton thought up The Money Man, a creative way of divesting himself of excess USA Distributors' cash, Jackie objected. Greedy fuck was too stupid to know that too much money meant too much scrutiny. What they needed was a way to get rid of money in a way that would both be completely underground and amusing. Recapturing the powerful feelings he first felt dealing drugs to the football players his father so deeply adored was a bonus. He never touched drugs himself—no, no, the high he got was from dealing and he needed it as much as the addicts needed their fix.

Communicating with terrorists was surprisingly easy, like plucking bad apples off the low branches of a laden tree. The most difficult part of the set-up had been finding a location where a gathering of international proportions wouldn't arouse suspicion. St. Bart's was perfect—sophisticated and very French, no one looked twice at his line of visitors, no matter how diverse, and Colton could conduct his business out in the open. The first time, he'd been nervous and cautious, afraid that every resort worker suspected the true nature of his business. He'd worked quickly back then, fearful of beggars. He'd dispatched them with efficiency and little dialogue, running down a written list prepared in advance, just to calm his nerves. As the word of The Money Man spread through the aggrieved communities of the world, many more began to show up. Now, he relished the power he wielded, and slowed the process a bit, enough to engage in some conversation with each one.

"Eight more outside, right?" he barked at Reggie.

"Eight more. Right," answered Reggie.

"Divide up the rest evenly and I'm done," said Colton.

Without waiting for a reply, he stood up and headed toward the door on the far side of the room. As he left the villa, he spied the Palestinian still struggling to move the heavy box of money out to a waiting car, and as Colton brushed by him, he tossed the earrings to the man, who said something, but Colton didn't bother to listen. Once he was gone, he knew the Palestinian would either have to get help quickly or divest himself of some of the cash in order to get it into his car, because Reggie, Gus, Stewart, and maybe even Hugh, led by Jackie, would steal some from him. If the others wanted to pocket some of the cash, it was theirs to steal, but only some, because Colton would hear if the man went away with nothing.

Once outside, Colton took a deep, long breath, cleansing himself of his morning and walked to the villa where Cherie waited. Exhausted from his morning business, he was now more interested in giving Cherie with the necklace. He needed a couple of drinks in him and to smell the luxuriousness of Cherie while he watched her stand before him wearing nothing but the necklace made from sacred gold.

Chapter 2

Form FDA 3500A, Incident #23:

There were three MIs on shift that night, about the same as any of regular shift. First one coded and we followed accepted procedure: begin CPR, administer clot busters, anticoagulants, and monitor heart activity. None of the common strategies worked with the first patient. We continued therapy with another round of meds to try to stabilize. In spite of continued therapy, patient did not respond at all and expired within minutes after therapy had begun. Upon review, the conclusion was that the patient presented in fragile condition, so initially we had no reason to suspect any issue with meds.

About an hour later, we took our second MI call. Second patient was also female, younger than the first. We followed the same accepted procedure, but again, no change in status. We administered a second round of medications and this time we did see some improvement, though not what we would have expected considering dosage.

Later than same night, we saw our third MI and saw the same results. Now we started to become suspicious of the medications. Expiration dates were within range, but we saved the empty vials from the three cases to see if they could be tested for content. Test results showed that the amount of drug in the sample was about half of what should have been in the vial. Turned it over to pharmacy after that…

***

Kat pulled the truck into the underground garage, grabbed her bag from the back and headed to the lobby to check in. There was something comforting about the good old Holiday Inn in West Philly. It was nothing fancy but was always the same. Always clean and predictable. It was the same feeling she got when she checked into the room and snapped the TV to CNN or QVC.

Kat plugged in her laptop and then got a hot shower going. She unpacked a few of her clothes and hung them up but was more interested in peeling off her clothes and hopping into the hot shower she missed in the morning's rush. Her best-laid plans had been scrambled first thing when Maryann called to tell her to report to the office for a special morning meeting to brief everyone on the Vioxx recall. So much for her house cleaning and all the other ritualized tasks she always did before leaving home. One of the joys of leaving was returning home to a spit and polish house—one that stood at attention in her absence, waiting for her return. This time she'd have to settle for a house at ease instead.

There was nothing out of the ordinary about the Vioxx recall—just standard stuff really—but the spotlight was on the division, so Dan took extra precautions to make sure all of his ducks were in a row. It was a highly charged political atmosphere and the department was issued a silent mandate to clamp down faster on offenders. After years of having his hands tied, Dan was taking his opportunities when he could, but he also knew he couldn't afford any mistakes or missteps. He was a pretty savvy guy, well aware that the manufacturers were going to pull out the big guns in response, so he made sure his department was thoroughly briefed and that everyone was working from the same handbook. While Kat was thrilled with the change in the department, this morning was an inconvenient time to have her routine interrupted. The more she studied her other cases, the more the Vioxx recall seemed like baby stuff by comparison.

She relished the steamy water pouring over her, working out the kinks from her drive and allowing her to concentrate on tomorrow's meetings with Blank and TemePhelps. She was always on guard at the on-site, always thorough, but this one was going to drag out. There were just too many unanswered questions. Her initial approach needed to set the tone for all future meetings and Kat wanted to make sure that these guys felt relaxed and comfortable. Contentiousness was the last thing she needed right now. Experience had taught her that the whole process slowed down if the manufacturers dug in their heels and pulled in the legal heavy hitters. It was a not-so-elaborate dance where everybody knew the steps and one that could get more tangled up than necessary if they got off on the wrong foot. Kat knew what she was entitled to see, they knew exactly what they were legally obliged to turn over, and everyone knew that if they didn't comply with her paperwork requests someone was going to jail.

After basking in her shower until she felt guilty, Kat finally exited, dried off, and called Jimmy Kirk, an old colleague who worked for a distributor in the area. Reps always had an ear to the ground and, for the right kind of flattery, were willing to divulge it. Kat had worked with Jimmy at Johns Hopkins fresh out of pharmacy school and the two became fast friends, a couple of times almost a little more, but somehow they were never single at the same time. They bumbled through their first few years as hospital pharmacists together, braving all the crummy shifts, the holidays, the on-call, and the abusive attendings. Kat liked Hopkins but Jimmy wasn't the kind of guy for the rigidity and rules of the hospital environment.

He took a spot at TemePhelps and moved up to Philadelphia. The sales game seemed perfect for him and every chance he got, he was calling to convince Kat to join him. Kat might have considered it but she had met Jorge and it looked like the two of them were headed down the aisle.

Kat kept up with Jimmy for most years but like with everything else in her life, she lost track when Jorge got sick, then just stopped trying to communicate with any more than her closest friends after he died. She hoped Jimmy would understand. He was no doubt a good "background" source in the investigation, somebody who might be able to fill in the personality stuff on the manufacturers. Good investigating was as much a matter of luck as it was preparedness and persistence.

Once dressed, Kat flipped open her cell phone and called Jimmy's number, hoping it had stayed the same after all these years.

"Jimmy? It's Kat Vasquez," she said.

"Hey, Kat! How the hell are you?" he answered. He sounded genuinely pleased to hear from her.

"Good. Good. How's with you?"

"I'm great! Things are really going well."

"So, I'm in Philly and I have a couple of hours to kill and I wondered whether I could buy you a drink. Catch up a little." She figured she'd get right to the point and move things along since she still needed to leave time for Albe and Martha later and it was already five o'clock.

"Either you're a psychic or you have great luck, but I'm just leaving a Center City appointment now. Where can I meet you?"

"You tell me and I'll get there."

"Well, hell, it's been a long time so let's do the Swann Lounge at the Four Seasons on the Parkway," he suggested.

"Sounds great. See you there in a half hour?"

"You got it."

Kat took one last look at her notes, then quickly got ready. It might be fun to catch up with him He was always that guy in the room, the one everyone wanted to know. Out of nowhere, Kat caught her thoughts quickly jumping from remembering back to dating days when she and Jimmy almost had a thing and tonight… She stopped short in the middle of the room. That was the first time she even imagined someone other than Jorge. She quickly shook it off, "the guy's married," she scolded.

Still, she dug through her suitcase, imagining that there was something more interesting in there to wear, gave up and finally settled on a standard pair of black slacks and a black and white patterned silk blouse. She tried to carefully apply what little make-up she had with her, stepped back from the mirror and stared. The makeup helped but her hair was still awful. She coaxed it this way and that, trying to make a style out of it, and finally found some old clips in the bottom of her case that she used to pull pieces back off her face and into some kind of vaguely deliberate design. She sighed, shook her head, and reached for her perfume. When all else fails, leave an alluring scent. Kat had always been partial to high-end classic French perfumes, now that was the only distinctive thing she had about her. She took in the scent, smiled vaguely, snapped off the bathroom light, and made her way toward her SUV.

Philadelphia had changed quite a bit in the last few years. The drive through the West Philadelphia area showed the University of Pennsylvania was more built up than before, looking more like a college town than a forgotten, run-down section of the city. She made her way over the Schuylkill River on the Spring Garden Bridge to get to the Art Museum circle, taken by how the lowering sun lit up the iconic Greek revival building on the hill. From there she looped onto the pride of the city, The Benjamin Franklin Parkway, one of the most beautiful parts of any city in the United States. Kat always tried to make it a point to walk the Parkway when she was in town, from the Art Museum at one end down to Logan Circle at the other. Considering the spectacular sunset, it seemed especially a shame to be too rushed to enjoy her favorite stroll. She made her way down the Parkway and around Eakins Oval, a series of three circular plazas, the centerpiece of which is an equestrian statue of General George Washington. Albe talked all the time about how college kids who got trashed and climbed up onto that statue to ride the horse with old George and Kat presumed he spoke from personal experience. Along the Parkway were most of the city's museums, including the new Barnes Foundation, home of the world's largest collection of post-impressionist art, the Philadelphia Free Library and tree-lined parks where crowds gathered for parades and concerts. It was also a short distance away from where a statue of William Penn surveyed the action from his perch atop City Hall. As she drove east on the Parkway, she could see Logan Square at the opposite end, one of the four squares included in William Penn's layout of Philadelphia. What most visitors knew about Logan Square was Swann Fountain, known as the Fountain of the Three Rivers, though they didn't always know that it was named for Dr. Wilson Carey Swann, founder of the Philadelphia Fountain Society and the swans in the water feature were in his honor. It was designed by sculptor Alexander Stirling Calder. The three Native American statues represent the bodies of water that snaked through the city, the Schuylkill River, the Delaware River and the Wissahickon Creek. But what Kat remembered about Logan Square is that in the early 1800s it was the site of public executions. Every time she was near Logan Square, she imagined the gallows still there being overseen by Billy Penn from his City Hall perch. For some reason the public executions intrigued her and she tried to envision what crime the offending party committed that netted them death by hanging. She envisioned Joel Klein hanging from gallows on Logan Square and wished for supernatural powers to meld the two times to make that possible. Kat reluctantly shook off the image as she pulled onto a side street and was lucky enough to find a metered parking place.

The Fountain Room at the Four Seasons had two-story high windows and Kat she peeked inside as she passed wondering whether Jimmy was there already. Would she even recognize him after more than a decade? She sincerely hoped he hadn't gotten too bald or too fat, then too, she hoped he wouldn't cringe at the sight of her.

"You look exactly the same," he said before she could get two feet into the Swann Lounge.

"You always were a good liar. But you really do look pretty much the same."

He was just a little thicker around the middle, but he still had the same gray eyes. He still kept his dark brown hair a little on the long side and now there was salt and pepper at the temples that complemented both his eyes and his crow's feet. They shared a long, warm hug, which felt more spectacular than she would have guessed. She stepped back and gave him the once over again.

"The years have been pretty good to you," she said.

"Well, outwardly maybe, but inside I've got that mid-life thing going on. You know, all the questions—where am I going? What's life really about? Heady stuff."

Kat closely watched his face before she reacted, unsure of whether she was hearing jokester Jimmy or another new Jimmy. His expression was somber so she scrambled for something to say to lighten the mood.

"Sounds like time to take a break from work and enjoy some time with Cathy, huh?" she said.

"I would, but her new husband might object," he shot back.

Kat felt the color rise in her cheeks.

"I'm sorry, I didn't—" she fumbled.

"Hey, no. No big deal. It was a big deal, financially and emotionally but there was nothing I could do about it."

Thankfully, the waiter appeared and took Jimmy's order for bourbon, straight, and a red wine for Kat.

"Long way from pitchers of lousy beer, huh?" she asked.

"I'm still happy with a pitcher of beer," he replied.

The waiter quickly reappeared with their drinks and they toasted before their first sips.

"I'm sorry," Kat offered after she swallowed. "I didn't know,"

"About Cathy? No, no, I knew you didn't know, so I told you. Figured I'd get it out of the way right off the bat," he said.

He closed his eyes as he took a long swig of his drink. She watched him until he opened his eyes again.

"Mind if I ask what happened?" she asked.

"Too many years on the road, I guess. I think I just stopped paying attention, you know? By the time I figured that out, she was done with me and now… anyway, it's amicable, for the sake of the kids. But now I want to talk about you," he insisted.

In spite of his words, Kat could hear the sadness in his voice but she knew better than to pursue that with him at the moment. It was startling to see this side of Jimmy, so different from the Jimmy she remembered.

"Jorge lost his battle with cancer about five years ago and since then, I left pharmacy practice and now I'm an investigator with the FDA."

He sat back in his chair and slammed down his glass, saying, "Wait, wait. That's too much for one sentence. Let's take this one at a time. What happened to Jorge?"

"Remember the headlines about the guy, Klein, who was diluting the chemo meds?"

"*That* jerk supplied Jorge?"

She nodded her head. Jimmy sighed heavily and shook his head.

"I feel like I should have known better, that's the thing. I should have been able to figure it out when the chemo wasn't making him that sick or tired. I should have known that it was because it wasn't working and not because he was so healthy or strong."

She fiddled with her wine glass; he reached across the table and patted her hand. She thought she felt a little spark but shook it off, embarrassed.

"You couldn't have known," he said.

"Thanks, but you and I both know I should have been suspicious," she croaked.

"Sounds like you just want to wallow," he replied.

She pulled her hand back, out of his reach, and sat back, a moment to process beyond her first reaction. He was right, of course. She was still carrying around the weight of her guilt like a badge. It was as though the guilt substituted for a portion of the grief, and as the grief subsided, the guilt was there to shelter her from moving on.

"I heard rumblings about that guy," Jimmy continued, easing the silence. "I was with TemePhelps at the time, but you hear things when you're traveling around. Some of the wholesalers mentioned certain guys who seemed to do a bigger business out the door than the supply they brought in the door."

"Not enough punishment in the world for guys like that," she said, taking a big swig of her wine.

"So, FDA, huh? You went over to the dark side," he offered, changing the subject.

"I'm the dark side?" she asked.

"Kidding," he laughed. Kat smiled.

"So, I heard you're a wholesaler now?" she offered.

"Partner in a distributorship. Yeah, a few of the guys were sick of the road and when GlobalMed came up for sale we pooled together and bought it."

"How big's your reach?"

"National, some international accounts. We've pretty much doubled the business in the past five years, but we're leveling off now."

He reached into his inside jacket pocket, pulled out a business card and slid it across the table.

"You seeing any increase in adverse reaction reports or efficacy complaints?" she heard herself way too eagerly.

"Any drug in particular?" he asked.

"Broad spectrum, number of different manufacturers," she replied casually.

"I'm not hearing about on my supply, but I'll keep an ear out."

Kat picked up the card, eyed it for a moment and slipped it into her handbag. She had to tread lightly here, picking at information without tipping too much of what she was working on. Even though some of the issues had already been picked up by the press, she didn't want to be the one spreading potentially harmful information when she didn't have all the facts lined up yet. She had to be especially suspicious of every manufacturer, every distributor, and every pharmacy until the source of the rash of recent MedWatch reports was traced.

"So, you have two girls, right?" she asked, changing the subject.

"Girl and a boy. Seven and ten. Shared custody with Cathy. It's working out okay for now. Funny, now I'm not on the road as much and I have a lot more time to spend with them, but it's too late."

He looked so melancholy that she had to stifle the temptation to want to take care of him.

"But Jimmy, aren't you the famous party guy? I would think you're out there living it up."

"I never thought I would say this, but it gets boring after a while. Philadelphia's a great place to meet women, but I'm getting too old for a lot of them."

"What?!" She tossed him mock surprise.

"What?" He seemed genuinely baffled.

"I didn't think it ever worked that way," she continued. "I didn't think guys ever thought they were too old or the girls were ever too young."

"Works that way for me," he answered in a far more serious tone than she would have liked.

"So, what about you? You dating?" he asked.

"Not even looking. Albe's at the University of Pennsylvania so I'm all alone in the house. It's pretty quiet, but I'm managing. Got a crazy dog that keeps me going sometimes."

Kat hated that this was turning into a lonely hearts meeting and she was itching for a way to get out of there. She glanced at her watch and saw that she had only been there for half an hour and supposed that it was probably still too early to meet Albe and Martha. College kids are on a schedule like Spain where they think 10 p.m. dinners are the norm. She searched for a way to wrap up the evening without hurting his feelings.

"You hungry? You doing anything for dinner?" Jimmy asked.

"I have to meet up with Albe and his girlfriend for dinner. I think this one's kind of serious," she said.

"That must be weird."

"Makes me feel old but then Albe says I should use it for an excuse to start looking for someone for me." The words came out before she hold them back. Now she struggled to keep the color from rising in her cheeks.

"You should be looking, Kat. You're smart, attractive, accomplished—"

"Enough of that. Anything you can tell me about TemePhelps or Blank?"

He sat back in his chair and raised his eyebrows.

"Oh, I get it. You're not interested in meeting up with an old friend. You're pumping me for information." He seemed more amused than annoyed.

"Just conversation…"

"Bullshit. I haven't forgotten how you could get just about anything out of just about anybody."

"Oh, well, Stacey Novak had it coming. She slept with the only hot intern of the bunch so we had to have details at least."

"Tell you what. We can talk some more over dinner sometime. I can fill you in on a lot of juicy details about the market here. How's that?" he offered.

Kat smirked.

"You win. Give me a call," she replied.

It wasn't the answer Kat really wanted but it was the answer that would get her out of the lounge right now. She finished the last sip of her wine and stood up to leave. Jimmy jumped up from his seat and enveloped her in a hug that Kat enjoyed more than reason told her to. She left him in the lounge nursing his second drink. Though he looked pretty much the same, Jimmy was very much a changed man. Either the years or his circumstances had calmed him down, made him the grown up he probably needed to be. But he sure wasn't the kind of company she remembered. No doubt he could be a valuable resource but the question was whether she could manage to be around him. The thought made her chuckle. She herself must have been enormously unappealing to be around for the first two years after Jorge and yet her friends hung in there with her. She probably owed Jimmy the same. Besides, she had a tough time forgetting that little twinge she felt just being around him.

After a quick phone call to Albe to firm up plans, she eased out of her parking spot and drove back to her hotel. Kat freshened up a bit at the hotel and waited for Albe and Martha, surprised at how nervous she felt. It was almost like she was going on a first date. She didn't have long to wait in the lobby before she spotted Albe with a lovely young woman by his side. She scolded herself for thinking it but she was relieved that he wasn't bringing some blonde bombshell, instead he walked in with a dark haired beauty who stood almost as tall as he did.

"Mom, this is Martha Famosa."

Martha reached out and shook Kat's hand firmly, and looked her right in the eye, confident, poised, and polite. As Kat smiled and exchanged niceties, she realized she really liked the girl already.

"So, I'm starving," Kat announced. "What're we eating?"

"Italian. Nice little place just down the next block," Albe replied.

The trio walked to the restaurant—three abreast with Albe between his mother and his girlfriend. Kat stole glances at him and felt her heart flutter as she noticed that he held hands with Martha. It would have been nice to be more prepared to meet his girlfriend. She was always frustrated with how secretive Albe was with his personal life, but then she supposed he'd rather wait until he was sure about something, before unleashing it on the Mom examiner.

They made it to the restaurant in just a few short minutes and were seated immediately. It was a family place but more sophisticated than the checkered tablecloth variety Italian restaurant. She ordered a nice bottle of wine to share, which arrived along with a crusty loaf of bread, fresh roasted peppers, and a dish of herbs and oil for dipping. There was little conversation while they decided on their entrees, but once everyone ordered, Kat turned her full attention to Martha. Albe rolled his eyes and waited for the onslaught of questions.

"So, Martha, are you from the Philadelphia area originally?"

"My family lives in South Jersey now, but my dad's originally from Mexico. Mom's local. Grew up on a chicken farm in South Jersey."

Kat glanced at Albe, who sat back in his seat and narrowed his eyes at her.

"Are they still in the chicken business?" she asked.

"Noooo. They own a restaurant in Cherry Hill, New Jersey. They're working on opening another one in Haddonfield soon."

"So, are you interested in going into the family business?"

She laughed and looked back at Albe, who changed his closed his eyes and put his head back. Martha cracked a smile and turned back to Kat.

"I'm afraid I'm not cut out for the restaurant business. I spent a lot of time there as a kid, but I guess I'm just sick of it."

"Martha's the first one in her family to go to college." Albe positively glowed when he made this announcement.

"Pretty impressive college for a first timer," said Kat.

"Oh, yeah. Thanks," she said shyly.

This girl was the perfect mixture of accomplishment and humility.

"What's your major?" Kat asked.

"At first I was pre-med, but honestly, I don't think I'm cut out for all the years of work that go into becoming a doctor."

"Well, you know…" Kat began.

"Oh, here it comes. Martha, don't say I didn't warn you," Albe said as he reached for a hunk of bread and his glass of wine. "Go ahead Mom, give Martha your spiel on pharmacy school. I've heard it dozens of times."

"Didn't work on you though, did it?" Kat said.

"Hey, finance is pretty darn respectable too, you know," he shot back.

Kat was struck by how much he looked like his father now, especially the way he moved his hands. She watched as he tore off a piece of bread and dipped it into the oil, using his left hand like his father. Jorge was the kind of guy who stuck with things, the kind who could always find another interesting angle to what he already knew. He had stuck with teaching for many years, and eventually moved to curriculum development, where he would have stayed until he retired if it weren't for Klein. Albe seemed only slightly like Jorge as a kid, but after he lost his father, he grew up fast, not that Kat needed him to but it was probably tough for him to have avoided it. Even without his father's guidance through his high school years, Albe kept a good head on his shoulders. Kat would have been proud no matter where he went but even she had to admit how proud she was when the acceptance letter came from the University of Pennsylvania. She had always thought that Albe would go into pre-med, and was surprised when he announced that he was majoring in business/finance.

"Mrs. Vasquez, Albe may not be interested in pharmacy school," said Martha, "but I am,"

Kat flashed a smile at Albe as he reached for more bread. Then she focused her full attention on Martha, talking up the virtues of becoming a pharmacist. Martha leaned in close and listened.

Kat sat back in her chair and added one last argument: "It's one of the few medical fields where women make up half the jobs and are equally compensated for their work. But it's also a field where there are a lot of highly compensated part-time opportunities that could fit into a parent's schedule." She finished with a half-hidden smile.

Kat glanced at Albe, then back at Martha, trying to detect some hint at the seriousness of their relationship, but neither betrayed anything, their expressions remaining blank.

"Okay, can we just eat now?" Albe asked.

On cue, the food arrived and Kat concentrated on the vodka salmon in front of her. She ordered a second bottle of wine for the table and began to unwind from a day that had more activity than she was used to.

"So Albe says you're an investigator with the FDA?" asked Martha.

"For the past few years."

"Working on anything interesting?" Martha continued pursuing more information than Kat was able to offer. Kat played with her wineglass deciding what to say.

"They're all interesting in their own way. Usually they turn out to be something small, but every once in a while we hit something big like the Vioxx case and it puts everybody on their toes," Kat said.

She almost convinced herself with her casual answer that the case she was currently working weren't huge, but she suddenly felt that familiar tingle down in her gut that snapped her back to reality.

"Yeah, I was reading about that Vioxx thing and it sounds like some kind of shady deal between the manufacturer and the FDA," said Albe.

"Nah, no deal. Just typical fast track approval. You're going to continue to see problems," she said. "Now, that's enough shop talk. Albe, I need a report on your classes."

She had downed one too many glasses of wine to risk talking in detail about her cases but not enough that she was reckless. Tomorrow she had site inspections at TemePhelps and Blank Products that would begin to reveal exactly what was causing the sudden rash of MedWatch reports and tomorrow would come soon enough. If she thought too long about how serious the problems could be, she might start focusing on the fact that the increased MedWatch reports might just the tip of the iceberg and that soon she would be inundated with cases, illnesses, and deaths. With little time and even fewer staff, she didn't want to imagine how she could even handle the worst.

***

Colton enjoyed his walk down the winding road, savoring the sunshine and the ocean breezes, shaking off the last few hours, anticipating his leisure time with Cherie. He passed through the gate to the private villa he'd enjoyed here for the past two years, pleased by the impeccable job his staff did of maintaining the grounds surrounding the villa and the pool and especially his orchid garden. Just the sight of his beloved gems puffed him up with pride. A smile crossed his face remembering the night at the snooty Philadelphia Orchid Society when he showed pictures of it by noted photographer Brian Ebers.

From the first time he came to St. Bart's, Colton was captivated by the fertile grounds. It reminded of when he was a kid spending hours at his mother's side learning the names of the plants, how to prune them in the fall and how to protect them in the winter. That was at the small house, the one they lived in when Daddy was the assistant coach at Michigan. That was before Daddy made the big time and they moved to Philadelphia, before he pronounced that no son of his would be some pansy digging up flowers in the garden. In the seclusion of St. Bart's far from his past, Colton could now be an indulgent gardener and orchids were his fascination.

He lingered for only a moment, before hurrying in to see Cherie. Inside, he brushed past the magnificent trays the staff always set up in the villa for his arrival—fresh fruits, cheeses, pastries, and even hand crafted chocolates, along with chilled champagne and a fully stocked bar-. The curtains to the terrace were drawn back to maximize the view and fresh towels, lightly scented with lavender, were piled on the chaise outside.

"Cherie?" he called to the empty villa.

Her voice floated to him from outside. "By the pool."

He could hardly contain his excitement. The sun was beginning to wane, the hottest part of the day retreated, and the shadows from the awnings covered a good portion of the pool deck. And there, in the shadows, perfectly golden from her earlier sunbathing, laid Cherie in a black bikini that was almost too small for her. It was the one for him, one that would never appear on the public beach.

"I have something for you," he said as he stepped out onto the back patio.

"How were your meetings? Are you terribly exhausted?" she asked.

He desired her more for that way she always asked about him first. She put down the book she was reading and curled her legs away from the end of the chaise, making a place for him to sit. Her lotion was vaguely coconut, maybe a bit buttery and tropically floral. The fabric of her bikini strained against her curves.

"I managed to get away from the meetings early enough and find this gift for you," he lied, holding out the velvet sack.

She sat up straighter on the chaise, cocked her head, flipped her raven hair and leaned over to accept the gift. But before she even opened it, she leaned over and kissed him, grateful for whatever it was. He savored the kiss and held himself back from pushing her down on the chaise and taking her right then.

"You're so thoughtful," she said.

"It's easy to be thoughtful with you," he said.

Before her, he would have strong-armed a woman to get his way, a pleasure he had learned early on from his father's "juiced" players. Choking was his favorite: he loved to see the marks on their throats and watch the redness as it rose up on their faces. He would keep one hand free so he could jam himself inside of them to come quick and hard. There were no better climaxes than that but then afterward they would cry or complain or just be afraid of him, and he hated that. He would convince them to stay, being nice to them for as long as it took to trust that they would keep quiet. Then they would leave. Did they really think he would hurt them? No, no, he was loving them, he insisted, loving them the best way he knew how. The whores taught him that he needed control these urges so as not frighten them away. Begin with patience— build trust, groom them, then maybe there would be the day he could do things his way. He watched Langford with Patricia, studied how he treated her and vowed that he would find his own Patricia.

"Colton, it's beautiful!" Cherie gushed as she pulled the necklace from the bag.

"I'm glad you like it. When I saw it, I imagined what it would look like on you. What it would look like if that was all you were wearing."

He watched her face as he delivered the line and knew immediately that she understood. That was another reason he truly loved Cherie. She undid the bra catch and pulled off her top her breasts falling into her waiting hands. Then she dangled the necklace from her left hand as she leaned toward him as she rose from the chaise. Coyly, with her back to him, she shimmied out of her bikini bottom to reveal her plump, round ass. She lifted the necklace as she watched him over her shoulder, when she turned around and showed her naked self to him, she was dressed only in the necklace made of sacred gold and blood red stones. He gasped. The sight of her was better even than he had imagined and stood to touch her. He felt as if he would explode. He wanted to hold on until he was inside of her, but she drew back and he was instantly annoyed at her. Then she smiled and he realized that she was teasing him, beckoning him to something even better. Her fingers caressed the necklace, lingering over each stone, playing with the pearl in the same way she played with him. He was mesmerized. She stepped backward, keeping her eyes on him and fingering the necklace while drawing him in to the bedroom. He followed. The necklace around her neck was like his hand, squeezing, as though each stone was the mark of a separate finger. She lay down on the bed and the necklace slipped up close to her neck and he gasped again, realizing that the Palestinian's gift was the perfect substitute for where he loved his hands to reside while he was in a woman. His orgasm was powerful, as powerful as before, and yet there was no danger is losing his Cherie. How could the Palestinian have known?

He lay down next to her and exhaled for a long time, letting go of all the toxic breath of the day. The sun was almost down now and the light in the room grew dimmer, lulling him off to sleep.

"You want to get some dinner?" Cherie asked softly.

Colton heard the words but translated them into his twilight dream. He tried to make sense out of the soft words that darted through his harsh conversation with a colleague. Cherie touched him gently on the arm and drew him out of his dream.

"What?" he barked, startled.

"Are you hungry? Do you want me to cook something?" she asked softly.

"No. No. We'll go out," he replied.

He was fully awake now and glanced at his watch. He'd been out for two hours, but the night was still young. There would be plenty of time for liquor, food, dancing maybe, and another round with Cherie.

"Let me get ready. I already took a shower while you slept. I was afraid I would wake you, but you were out like the dead," she said.

He winced. He hated expressions like that. He was about to scold her but she slipped off her towel and stepped into a flowing dress with spaghetti straps and a deep V plunge in the front. He instantly forgot his annoyance. He was disappointed when she pulled a pair of panties out of her suitcase and slipped them on. But he was cheered when she pulled a pair of lovely high heel sandals, tall and strappy, onto her feet. She was prettier than Langford's wife, prettier by far and probably much better in bed. One day he would be sure to confirm that. He made a note to watch Langford carefully the next time they were together to detect whether he also thought that Cherie was prettier than Patricia.

Colton rolled off the bed and changed into linen slacks and a silk polo shirt, and ran a comb through his thinning hair. He felt his face for stubble and half disappointed, half relieved, concluded that he didn't need to shave. His beard was soft and thin, like an adolescent boy's still to this day, and there were times it made him feel less virile if he allowed it. Today, he was able to ignore it. He finished dressing and waited for Cherie to join him at the front door.

They would go to the resort, where they knew him the best and stumbled over themselves to serve him. Sometimes in town the locals were not as impressed with him as they should be.

"Ready?" he called.

"One minute," she replied.

He called Reggie to bring the car around and waited until he pulled up in the rented Jaguar. Reggie jumped out to open the door for Colton just as Cherie joined them. Colton stepped back and allowed Cherie to enter the car first, then followed. Reggie slammed the door shut, then got in himself.

"Where to, Boss?"

"Eden Rock."

Reggie began to pull away until Colton hollered for him to stop.

"You're not wearing it," Colton said.

"What?" she asked.

"The necklace. You need to wear the necklace," he said.

"It doesn't go with what I've got on," she protested gently.

"Go put it on," he whispered quietly into her ear.

She smiled, then got out of the car and headed back into the villa. He watched her, then turned to Reggie and watched how he stared at Cherie's ass. He loved that Reggie lusted after his girl, loved it more that he would never have her. In just a few moments, Cherie re-emerged from the villa and made her way back into the car. He could see the necklace prominently around her neck. When she got inside, Colton ran his fingers over the necklace. He kissed her lightly on the neck, whispering, "Thank you" so only she could hear. She smiled, then turned her face away from him and looked out the window.

Reggie pulled out and expertly navigated the narrow winding streets until he pulled up to the front door of the five-star resort where a uniformed attendant opened the door and greeted them. Colton held out his hand for Cherie, then walked with her into the lobby and steered her into the dining room where the maître d' greeted him by name and hurried off to find them a table by a window. Once seated, Colton gazed out the window at the bay and the yachts he'd chartered.

"Let's go out on the water tomorrow," he said.

Cherie made a pinched face, then, with a faint smile, nodded.

"You don't want to go?" he probed.

"Maybe you'll have a lot of meetings again and be too tired. The water makes people tired," Cherie said.

He looked around the room and recognized the men eating dinner together. Most ignored him, remembering the strict orders issued to them that they were never to acknowledge him in public and never, ever, associate themselves with him. These men behaved. Why didn't Cherie?

"Why don't you want to go out?" he asked.

He studied the men around the room as she spoke, memorizing what they ate and drank, filing it away for future reference. The Africans liked brightly colored drinks, the Middle Easterners only hard liquor or tea; the Russians drank straight vodka and the Europeans stuck to wine and beer. He found out early that their drink preferences were no measure of their hardness.

"I didn't say I didn't want to go out," she said, laying her hand on his.

Colton looked at her, then past her to the corner of the room where he noticed the Palestinian who gave him the necklace sitting all alone and gazing out the window. This old man was eating only a bowl of soup, probably the cheapest thing on the menu, and nursing a glass of strong tea. Either Reggie and the others had stolen too much of his money or this was a man of scruples who would not squander the resources meant for his organization. Colton liked him when he first came, not just because of the necklace, but because he was too old for this game and still had the courage to play. For once he wanted to know a real name, to know something more about one of these men. He motioned to Reggie, who was standing by the door of the restaurant.

The waiter got to the table before Reggie and delivered a white wine for Cherie and a glass of hundred-year-old Aberlour a'bunadh Scotch whiskey, neat, for Colton. He placed them on the table without a sound. Colton savored the first sip of Scotch as the smoky goodness washed over his tongue and burned the entire way down to his stomach. He realized that he had been waiting for liquor all day.

Reggie stood patiently waiting by the table. Colton ignored him for now and savored another sip while regarding the Palestinian. He pondered whether he should send for the man so he could see the necklace on Cherie.

"What do we do instead, Cherie?" he asked suddenly.

She looked up from her glass, startled, and fumbled for an answer.

"Hmmmm. I don't know."

"You don't want to go out of the water, but you don't have any other plans instead," he said.

He had been growing impatient, but the Scotch began to have an effect on him. He watched the Palestinian. The man had finished his soup and tea and was paying for them with a handful of coins that he plopped on the silver tray where most others flipped a credit card.

"You guys take everything I told him was his?" he asked Reggie.

"I'm going to the ladies' room," said Cherie, rising from her seat. She brushed past Reggie on her way past.

"You want me to go with her?" he asked as she left.

"You guys take everything?" Colton repeated, ignoring Reggie's question.

Reggie shifted from one foot to the other before answering.

"Fifty, right?"

"That's what I said. What did he actually get?"

Reggie hesitated, shifted, fell silent, then finally answered.

"A little less."

"How much less?"

"Not too much."

Colton knew he was making Reggie sweat. If they took too much from the Palestinian, he would issue an order to get a message to the man to come back again in three months and collect more funds. In the meantime, he would make Gus or Stewart pay for the mistake in front of the others, just as a reminder.

"Should I ask him how much he got?" Colton asked.

As he said this, the Palestinian stood up from his seat and walked toward the door. He tossed a quick glance at Colton, then straightened his gaze out to the lobby beyond the restaurant. Colton shifted in his seat to watch the Palestinian leave, though he made it look as though he was casually looking around the restaurant. The view to the lobby was clear; the Palestinian stopped abruptly to greet Cherie. Then, he pointed at the necklace. Cherie smiled broadly at whatever he said and blushed a little. The man handed her something and Colton could see that she was hesitant to accept, but she took the item nonetheless, before making her way back to the table.

Colton watched the Palestinian scuffle out of the lobby and out of his sight. This man intrigued him. He should have been a man at an age to enjoy his life and his family, to enjoy the rewards of his many years of struggle, but he was still unsettled and spending his time meeting with The Money Man and collecting funds that would be used to kill those he hated. Or maybe not. Maybe he was a better con man than the others and an international jewel thief, perpetrator of the perfect crime by stealing from The Money Man by posing as a terrorist. Colton actually liked the idea of this. He turned his attention to Cherie.

"What did he say about the necklace?" he asked.

"Who?" she replied.

"The old man you spoke to out there. What did he say about the necklace?" Colton pressed.

"Something about sacred gold and blood red stones. I didn't like what he said," Cherie replied.

Colton eyed Cherie closely. Her fingers were busy fiddling with her drink.

"He might have been a good man," he offered.

"Do you know him?" she asked, looking up at Colton.

As soon as she asked the errant question, she clamped her mouth shut and apologized. Colton forgave her immediately, but only because he had now finished half of his Scotch. He surveyed the room to see how many of the other men were still there and counted ten he recognized.

"He also handed these to me," she said as she placed the earrings on the table between them.

He scooped up the earrings and slipped them into his pocket, annoyed at the Palestinian. Maybe his mother would enjoy them instead.

"Are you ready to order?" the waiter asked. The maître d' rushed over to the table and shooed the waiter away.

Colton turned his head to hide his amusement at his panicked face.

"I am so sorry Mr. Barnes. He is new here and I'm afraid I did not train him properly. Chef will have your meals prepared quite soon," gushed the maître d'.

Colton nodded at him kindly while enjoying his panic, then turned his attention back to the men in the room. Now he thought it should be required of them to bring him gifts. Why shouldn't they?

"Tell them I want gifts," he said suddenly to Reggie.

"Gifts?" Reggie asked.

"Next time. They should bring gifts," Colton repeated.

"Ah, what kind of gifts?"

"Tell them to ask the Palestinian."

Reggie looked baffled but said nothing more. Let Jackie and Hugh explain it to Reggie. Colton drifted off, imagining what gift he could expect and entertained himself with thoughts of jewels, animals, antique liquors and exotic cars. It would be fun to see how creative they got.

Dinner arrived. Colton finished his Scotch and asked the sommelier to bring a bottle of fine French wine to accompany the food. The man scampered away as if on a cloud, which made Colton laugh. He plowed into his filet mignon with relish, and after a partial belly full of food and a glass of exquisite wine, he regarded Cherie again.

"How is your fish?" he asked.

"Delicious. The best yet," she replied with a smile.

She said what he wanted to hear, but he watched her push the food around on her plate. She had developed this trick to prevent him from complaining about how she never ate. At first he watched her fork then focused his gaze on her breasts and back up to the necklace. She had been right; it really did clash with what she wore. But the sight of it stimulated him and he touched her foot with his under the table. She smiled at him and picked up her wine glass with both hands, the way he loved, sipping at the contents and keeping her gaze on him.

"So you don't want to go out on the water tomorrow," he said.

"I just thought that I may have gotten too much sun and being out on the water is really hard on your skin—"

"So, you don't want to go?" he pushed.

"No, Cole, sure I want to go," she purred.

She stroked his hand and smiled.

"You don't really want to go," he persisted.

"I'll just slather on sun block and wear a T-shirt. It'll be great," she replied.

He surveyed the room to see whether the men were noticing the affection he was receiving from a ravishing beauty.

"Good. We'll go in the morning," he finished.

Their dinner plates were whisked away now, replaced by desserts for each and steaming hot coffee. Colton usually had brandy with his coffee, but none appeared this evening and he wasn't in the mood to complain. Cherie attacked her dessert like it would run away if she didn't gobble it all down.

Suddenly, Reggie bolted from Colton's side, sprinted across the restaurant and tackled a man who shared a table with two other men and an older woman. As Reggie pummeled the man on the floor, the two men at the table jumped back but did not approach Reggie. The woman at the table screamed. The other diners reacted to the commotion-several women shrieked and a few men reached inside their pockets- and some diners didn't react at all, continuing to eat their dinner as though nothing were happening. Cherie gasped and partially hid under the table.

Colton watched Reggie pummel the man who now lay on the floor until he was unconscious while his dinner companions sat frozen in their seats, oddly silent, neither defending their companion nor making any attempt to prevent Reggie from completing his mission. Reggie scrambled back up to his feet and surveyed the room, then stepped back from the man on the floor. Around the room, the men who had registered the violence resumed eating or turned their gaze to the view out the window as though nothing had happened.

The maître d' approached Reggie and spoke, then snapped his fingers at the staff and two of the bigger waiters hesitantly stepped toward Reggie and the man. They helped him stand the man up and then stood back as Reggie escorted him out of the building. Colton waited for a moment before rising from his seat and holding his hand out for Cherie to take. She joined him and he stood next to the table for a moment, making eye contact with everyone in the room. In turn, they offered small responses, acknowledgements, and gestures of respect. Finally, he steered Cherie away from the table and out of the room.

After managing his crew in Camden for so many years, he knew that the look around the room was an important gesture. It was how a leader handled his pack of dogs and it was how he maintained his position without resorting to violence.

Reggie waited for them in the car alone. There was no sign of the man. Colton opened the door for Cherie. She rushed inside and Colton nestled in beside her as she threaded her arm through his and held tight. She was shaking. He immediately wanted to take care of her, comfort her, reassure her that everything would be okay. This was her first exposure and he sincerely hoped that she would stay with him.

"You're alright," he said, stroking the side of her face. She burrowed in closer to him.

He caught Reggie's eye in the rear view mirror and slightly nodded. Reggie tipped a finger to his forehead, driving them back to the villa.

When they pulled up, Reggie opened the door and the two exited the car.

"You go on ahead, love. I'll be there soon," Colton said to Cherie.

She hesitated. Then, she walked to the front door, turning to take one last look before she went inside.

"What was it?" Colton asked.

"Gun. Nothing big, maybe he wasn't even going to use it, but I made for a good display," Reggie replied.

"He was a nice choice. Central to the room and everyone got a good view. Good job."

"Maybe not the biggest guy in the room, but I thought he was a good mark. Played well with her, huh?" Reggie nodded toward the villa.

"We'll see. I hope it didn't play too well," said Colton.

He smiled at Reggie, who grinned in return. Then Colton squarely faced Reggie. He was roughly half his size and a lot less conditioned, but he used what he did have to get an answer out of Reggie.

"I still need an answer on the Palestinian's money," Colton said flatly.

Reggie began to speak, but hesitated. Colton drew closer, arms poised at his sides.

"We just took enough so that he could get the box into the car," Reggie said.

"Oh, so you helped him out, huh?" Colton shot back.

"Boss, we—"

Colton relaxed his arms, shoved his hands into his pockets and lifted his chin.

"I like him. I like the Palestinian. Next time he keeps everything," he said.

Colton turned and started toward the house, then paused and returned. He reached his arm out and Reggie flinched slightly. Colton clapped him on the shoulder and said, "Good work." He walked to the front door of the villa.

Today was a good day, better than he thought it would be. Tomorrow he would enjoy going out on the water with Cherie and relaxing in the garden. Then it would be time to head back to Philadelphia, back into his role of Owner/President of USA Distributors. Like a victorious general returning from war, he would march back into Philadelphia.

Chapter 3

Form FDA 3500A, Incident #131:

...Eighty-year-old female patient in cardiac intensive care being treated for congestive heart failure. Fluid level was accumulating around the heart and filling her lungs. Lasix treatment was begun. Usual dosing did not yield significant results so an additional course of treatment was prescribed, still without significant result. Lungs were drained and fluid removed and additional courses of Lasix were maintained, although with little result. Limited results were charted in 100 percent of cases where use of Lasix was clearly indicated and yet the use of the drug yielded little or no result.

Patient blood was drawn to check for levels and little or no drug was detected in the blood stream even after several doses were administered. Vials were isolated and returned to manufacturer for study and an FDA report was filed...

***

Kat always liked Charlie Sullivan at TemePhelps. He was a fuzzy teddy bear, a straight talker, bottom line kind of guy, who Kat honestly believed would never steer her wrong. She'd also been on enough inspections to know that guys like Charlie, no matter how nice, are pros. They reveal only what they must, answer only specifically what is asked, and fiercely protect their jobs. She could trust him, more than some others, but she knew to never really trust anyone completely.

"Well, look who blew up over the Mason-Dixon line," said Charlie as he shook her hand.

Drug companies were well acquainted with FDA inspections and their employees were well versed by highly compensated lawyers and consultants on how to handle them. Rule number one: be nothing but cooperative. Kat's first inspection with Charlie was two years ago and since then she'd been back three times, enough to be able to recognize changes in Charlie or his demeanor. Getting to know something about these guys personally wasn't just a formality. It was an important tool in recognizing when something was off. Might be something personal; then again, maybe not. Charlie looked as good as he did a year ago, with no hint of nervousness, no sign that he'd been under any kind of additional stress.

"Good to see you, Charlie," she said sincerely.

"You'll need these," he said, handing over security credentials. "C'mon back to the conference room."

Kat followed him down the hallway.

"How's that boy of yours?" he asked over his shoulder.

"Doin' well. Second year at Penn. Living at the frat," she replied.

"I remember those days… whew! I think I'm lucky that I do remember those days," he said.

"Oh, now, that's not what a mom wants to hear!"

He laughed and shrugged.

"How's your brood, Charlie?"

"Growing fast. Two teenagers now and all that goes with that."

They continued to chat as she followed him across the lobby, past the receptionist, down a short hallway and into a conference room befitting a multi-billion dollar international corporation. A petite young woman dressed in a lovely pink suit waited for them. She would be the scribe for the day, someone who would record every conversation Kat had with every employee in the facility.

"This is Louise, my assistant," Charlie said.

Kat nodded at the girl and smiled. Charlie waited for Kat and Louise to take seats, closed the door, and took up a chair across the table from Kat, waiting for her to speak. They both knew full well that when the door closed, the small talk was over and now their every word would be strictly business.

"Here's the 482 'Notice of Inspection' and I'm guessing you don't need to see my credentials, but here they are anyway." Kat pulled paperwork out of her case and placed it on the table.

Charlie pulled the notice and the credentials toward him. He examined them as a formality, an acknowledgement that Kat had offered them so that Louise would record it in her notes.

"After the on-site I need the logs, quality testing, contamination testing, and all other paperwork from the past six months," Kat said evenly.

She delivered her lines casually, trying to make him think the visit was strictly routine, but she was also gauging his every nuance. They both knew this visit was more than just routine; the timing alone should have clued him in. Manufacturers relied on the fact that the department was understaffed and couldn't get to field locations often, so getting visited only a few months after an inspection was a definite tip off. Kat watched Charlie, soaking in his every word and move. Kat was very good at was gauging sincerity. Years of practicing pharmacy in tough neighborhoods where addicted drug seekers were common made for good training on how to make accurate snap judgments. As much as she liked Charlie, she had to put that aside and bore in. It was an investigator's hard lesson learned that the very person you may not suspect is the very person you should.

"Okay if the plant manager takes you through while I get the logs, or do you want me for the day?" he asked.

"The plant manager's fine," she replied.

It was refreshing to work with a seasoned manager like Charlie and not having to waste time with bullshit. A less experienced manager would have suggested a PR pro or someone from the marketing department to accompany her through the facility. Kat was glad to not have to waste time waiting for an escort who could answer real questions. Everyone was supposed to know that when the FDA showed up, it was time to get serious. Charlie's job today was to make sure the FDA's on-site interactions were with only the most qualified and knowledgeable members of the company team. There were times Kat felt genuinely sorry for guys like Charlie, knowing full well that her appearance shoved them into the heart attack zone, even if they really had nothing much to worry about. Inspections always turned up something, usually something minor, but these guys had to answer for whatever she wrote up in her findings. She also knew if there was a problem going on, it generally wasn't with these guys; it was with whoever was spinning data or cutting backdoor deals or bringing in adulterated raw goods. Still, this was the way in the door and these were the guys who wouldn't hide the truth. They were also the first ones fired if she found something.

"I'll call over to him to get you started and set up whatever you need to see here in the conference room. Louise will be available for any copying you need done," he said.

"Thanks, Charlie."

He headed for the door, paused before he opened it and said, "Manager's name is Suresh Siddari."

"Thanks. Make sure you have all the 3500s you've gotten in the past eighteen months too." She said this casually, as though there were nothing unusual about her request.

"No problem.".

Charlie knew better than to ask what she was looking for, but he also knew she only usually asked for the past six months. Right now, he was probably going to look at the FDAs MedWatch 3500 forms while she was tied up in the plant and get an inkling of what she was up to before the inspection was over. He was going to call the corporate lawyers and let them know she was on site and have them pore over the 3500s and the FDA's log of recent inspection sites to see if this inspection was routine or whether it was something they needed to be concerned about. If they had something they underreported, they would be scrambling to get their stories straight. If there was something they were hiding, they were rushing the big guns over to the site to meet with her. But if they had nothing to hide, they were going to be as stumped as she was, because the reports were all over the place and the data inconsistent.

"Very pleased to meet you, ah, Miss Vasquez?" said Suresh as he and Charlie returned to the conference room.

Kat stood up and shook Suresh's hand, which was dripping with sweat. Poor guy was nervous. Could be because it was his first investigation or maybe he knew something. Kat studied him up and down and assessed him as young and scared, for now. She tried to be polite and not wipe her hand off and instead shoved it into the pocket of her slacks. Must be his first inspection, she thought.

"So, shall we get started?" she asked, picking up her case from the chair next to her.

They entered the plant through the door on the loading dock, just as the raw materials would in the manufacturing process. Louise followed along with her trusty notepad and pen. The manufacturer was responsible for the chain of custody on the drug—that is, providing a paper or electronic pedigree on the drug from raw materials to sale to a distributor. The distributor, in turn, was responsible for the drug's pedigree from manufacturer to drugstore, hospital or home care provider shelves. She expected Charlie to present logs representing each and every lot of raw material delivered to the plant in the past 18 months, and every process by which the raw material was combined into a finished form, tablet, capsule or injectable. She removed a number of sterile vials from her case and retrieved a sample of each raw powder in the area, under Suresh's watchful eye. She would have them tested by her lab and verify the testing results from TemePhelps. If they were deliberately bringing in substandard or contaminated raw goods, it would be found in testing.

Kat watched as the powders were offloaded into huge hoppers in the compounding area. Assuming the goods were clean, the next opportunity for adulteration or contamination was in the compounding area. She watched the delivery and everything appeared as it should. She checked off on her list that she didn't see anything that might be cause for contamination concern. She made eye contact with each of the workers and smiled. Connecting with every worker on-site indicated that she was open to being approached if anyone had anything she needed to hear. She knew from experience that if you give them an opportunity, someone always talked. Everyone here seemed contented and efficient. Kat moved on.

"Shall we suit up?" she asked, indicating that she was finished in the delivery and loading area and wanted to proceed to sterile production.

Suresh took her to the anteroom where the two of them put on "bunny suits," Tyvek outer suits that were used to cover up street clothes in the sterile area. She slipped the cap over her head and pulled the booties on over each of her shoes then finally donned the safety glasses before signaling that she was ready to go. Suresh pushed the button and the doors to the sterile area opened automatically. Kat followed Suresh in, with Louise and her notebook close behind. She took note that the workers in the area were properly suited and gloved and wore head coverings, safety glasses, and masks over their mouths. She checked to see that lots were being marked before production and properly labeled and quarantined after the product was finished. All the paper documentation would be waiting for her in the conference room, but for now, she was checking to witness proper procedure in the compounding area. She watched a technician pull out samples from the production, and then label and pack them to send to testing. Another technician came into the area and retrieved the samples to walk them down to the testing area.

"Testing?" she asked quickly. She wanted to see how the samples traveled at every step.

Suresh led her to the testing lab where the samples were unloaded, logged and left on a cart to be retrieved by one of the lab technicians who would perform the testing. There hadn't seemed to be an opportunity for any tampering with the samples before they got to the testing area, nor any way that the lab technicians could switch or enhance samples once they were in the area. Of course, as Kat well knew, anything is possible for someone who really wants to put his or her mind to it. The rash of MedWatch reports indicated that the scope of the occurrences was far larger than a single technician at a single facility; it would have to be a lot of technicians and a lot of forged testing results. She watched the technicians work under the Laminar flow hoods to maintain sterility. They then left the hood and used a rack-mounted laptop to record the results. She made a mental note to inquire about their Information Technology operation. The samples were then placed in a plastic tray, labeled, and stored on shelving in the next room, carefully organized so that they could be checked after the proper quarantine period and the lot could be released for shipment and sale. Kat was watching for the opportunity to fake the testing in some way, either by using pure product as sample rather than the actual product that was offloaded and for now. A supervisor, perched behind a glass window, surveyed the technician's work as well as verifying that their entire workday was recorded by a series of cameras positioned around the lab. If results were being tampered with or faked, it would have to be with the cooperation of the supervisor.

"Tableting area?" Kat asked.

Suresh nodded and ushered her back into the anteroom where they removed their bunny suits and left the building altogether. They walked through a maze of outdoor walkways under the overhead steam pipes before arriving at another building where the solid dosage forms were being produced. Again, Kat followed Suresh in through the loading area first and then inside the facility, with Louise close at her side. The machinery here was much louder than the sterile products area and Suresh encouraged her to wear ear protection as they suited up again. She watched as huge hoppers dispensed measured amounts of powder into a large mixing bin and began to stir the active ingredient together with various fillers, colorings and silicates until the correct formula for the drug was incorporated together. Then that mixture was poured into the elaborate machinery that would feed the powder through a die unique to the form of that tablet and exert the correct amount of pressure to properly form the tablet. Too much pressure and the tablet would move through the body and exit, unable to dissolve and unable to deliver the dose of the drug needed. Too little pressure and the tablet was too fragile and powdery, falling apart during shipment.

TemePhelps made both the name brand and the generic equivalent of their drugs in this facility, and while the active ingredient was exactly the same, the tablets were vastly different in color and shape. They would all be produced from many of the same raw ingredients and she knew to look on the MedWatch forms to determine whether similar complaints were found in both generics and name brands. Most of the solid dosage process was automated, although there were attendants on the floor to watch the machinery for proper function and shut down the line if necessary. Many manufacturers split up the process, using one facility for synthesis and another for manufacture, but TemePhelps had sunk a lot of money into this plant recently and were able to complete synthesis, purification, drying, milling, and storage of drug on this single site.

Kat continued through the facility, ticking off in her head what she expected to see along the way and taking note where there might have been a lapse in procedure or an opening for contamination. She didn't expect to see much out of line here, but the physical tour helped cement a snapshot of the production process in her head. As days went by, she knew questions would occur to her, questions that might be answered in the logs or questions that might nag at her and offer some clue as to what might explain the reports they were receiving. She removed some small envelopes from her case and retrieved some of each of the pills from the bins in which the machinery dropped them. Like vials, she clearly labeled and dated each envelope and slipped them all back into her case.

"Everything looks good from here," she said to Suresh, who visibly relaxed.

"Conference room?" he asked.

"Somewhere I can get a bottle of water too?"

He jumped into action, hurrying her back to the main building and the conference room before disappearing and reappearing with a bottle of water and a big grin. Kat thanked him and was tempted to pat him on the head for a job well done. He left the room and she chuckled. That this was not the type of guy who could survive doing anything compromising; whatever fell under his perusal would most certainly be on the up and up. Now she had to scrutinize the paperwork in front of her and find some clue as to what might be happening to TemePhelp's medications that warranted a rash of MedWatch reports.

She thought back to Dan and the first reports bad Heparin reports. The reports began to trickle in early 2007 but seemed too few to spot a trend. In a normal year, there would be about one hundred allergic reactions to Heparin, out of an almost one million doses administered each year. Suddenly in 2007, that one hundred jumped to three hundred and fifty, including nineteen deaths. Brad was already working the case when the number jumped and Dan immediately called a meeting to pore over the cases and make a decision as to whether all product should be recalled immediately. He paced the room, ranting, more heated than Kat had ever seen him, and with good reason. Though no one would say it out loud where the public could hear it, all the evidence pointed to deliberate adulteration rather than accidental contamination.

"Sloppiness or arrogance," Dan shouted. "Either way, these guys are not getting away with it!"

This was the beginning of a new age for the drug industry. For all of their policies and procedures and for all of the FDA's regulations and inspections, the world market and the constant quest to squeeze out one more penny of profit would eventually result in increased vulnerabilities. Not to mention that at the current rate, overseas facilities would only be inspected once every fifty years. A few weeks later, when Brad returned from China and issued the findings, they were more shocking than anyone would have guessed.

"The production of Heparin is sub-jobbed out to families in the rural areas of China, who have little regard for sanitary production methods. More ominously, with the increased prosperity in China, many of these families are able to send their children to the West for education, an education that can sometimes result in an increased knowledge of substances that may be used as cheaper substitutes and serve to adulterate the product and increase profitability. In the case of Heparin, over-sulfated chondroitin sulfate was added to increase the yield by anywhere from 5 to 20 percent. The chondroitin sulfate, made from animal cartilage, is structurally similar to Heparin and was deliberately used because the molecule bore such a close resemblance to heparin. It fooled standard quality tests and made it into the United States drug supply."

By the time Brad completed his report, Dan's face was red all the way down his neck and he was pacing the back of the room, periodically pounding on the wall. It was good that the FDA had someone like Dan in charge, someone who would take every violation of FDA regulation as a personal affront.

"When the hell's the meeting with the sub-committee?" he boomed.

"Tomorrow," answered Lee.

"Those guys need to grow a pair and give us something to work with here!"

Kat couldn't help but think about Jorge and shudder at the thought of a more organized group of counterfeiters willing to risk the lives of others for a mere increase in profit. The Heparin incident was a huge wakeup call; since then inspections had been stepped up substantially and Dan was busy hiring more inspectors to join the ranks. Meanwhile, reports on a number of other drugs began to trickle in and there was a kind of buzz around the department as if they were just seeing the beginning of what could turn out to be something frightening and huge. For the sake of the investigation, Kat had to keep an open mind, but deep down where her demons lived, she worried for every single American who was dependent on every single dose of medication and how many would be injured or die.

"May I bring you anything else?" asked Suresh, startling Kat and bringing her back to the present.

"Thanks. Any word on when Charlie is bringing the paperwork to me?" she asked.

"I'll check," Suresh replied.

He scampered out of the room and Kat checked her watch. She had already been there half of the day and it looked like she would probably have to return tomorrow. That meant her inspection at AmPharm would have to be shoved to the next day, which also meant Bernie needed to spend yet another day with Albe at the frat house.

She excused herself from Louise, saying she had to make a personal phone call, left the conference room and walked down the hallway. She clicked Albe's speed dial button on her cell phone.

"Hey, how's Bernie today?" she asked.

"He's fine," Albe replied.

He sounded like he just got up, which made Kat worry that poor Bernie spent the morning huddled in a corner, crossing his legs, trying not to pee in the house.

"I'm probably going to have to stay at least another day, maybe two. Is that okay for Bernie to stay on or should I find a kennel?" she asked, already knowing the answer.

"Mom, stop worrying. Bernie's fine. In fact, he loves it here," said Albe.

Kat had mixed emotions when she heard that, glad that he was happy there, worried that he would be sad to leave the party house and return with her to Maryland.

"You wanna grab something to eat tonight?" she asked.

"Can't. Midterms are next week and I've got to get a jump," he replied.

She bit her tongue so she wouldn't express her disappointment. It was harder to be close to him geographically but not be able to see him than it was to be back in Maryland. This was when she wished that she and Jorge had had more children. She banished that thought as quickly as it came. There had been enough pain around losing Jorge— she didn't want to revisit all the almost babies, the two miscarriages and one stillbirth that she and Jorge had hoped would be their expanded brood.

Kat snapped her phone shut and went back to the conference room to sit and wait for her paperwork, though she didn't have to wait long.

"Sorry for the delay," Charlie said as he entered a moment later with his arms full of binders.

He placed the binders on the conference room table and took a seat across from Kat, waiting for the questions. She opened her notebook with the 3500s inside and began. The description of the first case was really rather gruesome and she had debated long and hard before coming today whether to present it first. In the end, she decided that the gravity would be useful in flushing out any sign of premeditation from these guys.

"You read the 3500s I guess," she began, voice carefully measured. "Twenty-six separate cases of anaphylaxis with the anti-inflammatory alone. All the patients had no prior history of reaction to the drug. What can you tell me?"

Kat watched him carefully.

"We've looked at everything on our end and can't isolate anything that belongs to us. The raw materials testing showed up nothing out of the ordinary, and the lot testings were consistent," he said evenly.

All of what he said was easily verifiable. She pulled out her briefcase with the lot testing results previously obtained from TemePhelps and set about to match them with the ones Charlie had just brought with him. He waited, patient and silent, while she pored over the numbers on each of the reports and found them completely the same. Even the reports themselves were clearly copies of one another, with hand written notes that were exactly the same. So if the data wasn't falsified and the materials were verified as consistent, where was the problem?

She looked up at Charlie and asked the next question: "Are you in charge of hiring in the loading/shipping area?"

"Paul James runs that department," he said.

"He available?" she asked.

"I'll be right back," he replied.

Kat continued to go over the logs and reports in front of her. Nothing in any of the numbers caught her attention particularly. There were no spikes. Nothing seemed out of place. No sign of perfect numbers, which could indicate perfect duplication, which in turn might indicate falsification. The facility was certainly clean and efficient. There seemed to be little opportunity for contamination in pre-manufacturing or manufacturing. So, if something were happening, it was either in those raw materials or after the product was finished and ready to ship. She knew that was a matter of digging for personnel issues.

Charlie returned with an older black gentleman. James was a little rough around the edges and clearly annoyed that he was interrupted from his job today. Kat shook his hand, which was rough and calloused, and motioned for him to sit down with her.

"You want me here or out?" Charlie asked quickly.

"I prefer to meet with Mr. James alone," she replied.

Charlie exited the room while Kat and Mr. James settled into their seats. Louise was still busily recording everything that was happened and every word that was uttered.

"How long have you been the head of loading and shipping?" Kat asked.

"Head? Well, that's been about almost ten years. Before that I was workin' in the department for the last fifteen years," he said.

"So, you've been here a long time," she offered.

"Started as a temp worker, doing all the cleanup work in the warehouse," he said with a proud note in his voice.

Mr. James sat bolt upright, formal, attentive, with his hands folded on the table in front of him.

"You take great pride in your work here," she said as she smiled at him.

He did not return the smile.

"I like my job. Like the company. Look forward to retiring with some money in my pocket." He spoke evenly, measured.

"So, as the department head now, you have how many employees working for you?" she asked.

"Sixteen, full time," he said.

"You hired them all?" she asked.

"I hired a lot of them. Some been here since I've been here," he said.

Kat pretended to leaf though some paperwork in front of her, spinning her next move. Mr. James was silent, still. Kat sat back in her chair and began again.

"Tell me about your best employee," she said.

"I got a lot of good guys workin' over there," he said slowly.

"Anyone not so great?" she asked.

Mr. James hesitated. He bore into her and took his time before answering. Kat plastered a pleasant look on her face and waited.

"A couple," he finally said.

He was reluctant to answer the last question, suspicious of her and ever loyal to his guys. That might be a good sign that his department was clean or it could be a sign that he's in too tight with them and altogether there're in on something. Now she needed to move systematically and see where she got a rise out of him.

"Tell me about the not-so-great guys," she said leaning forward and resting her elbows on the table.

"Nothing much to tell," he shot back quickly.

"Mr. James, do I need to remind you that not being wholly forthcoming with me has some pretty bad consequences?"

He pursed his lips, pulled his hands off the table and rested them in his lap. Kat took it to mean he understood.

"Maybe if you tell me what you think is going on, I can help you," he said.

"Doesn't work that way, Mr. James. I ask, you answer. Then I draw a conclusion. Now, do you know anything about your guys and their personal lives?" she asked.

He looked at her a long time, squinted, and sized her up before answering.

"Some," he said.

"Anybody on the ropes? Nasty divorce, gambling problem, money problems, drugs, drinking… Anything like that?" Kat asked.

"Everybody's got something going on, but not on my time," said Mr. James.

"Something big enough to drive them to do something here that they shouldn't?" she asked quickly.

"I got cameras on every single one of them and everywhere else in the area, all day, every day," he said, losing his carefully measured tone. "If somebody was doing something, I'd know about it. Ain't none of my guys goin' to get away with doin' somethin' I don't know about. They know who I am. They know what kind of boss I am. Ain't none of my guys goin' get away with doin'somethin' I don't know about!"

Paul James convinced Kat right then. There was no conspiracy between him and someone else in the area, and without James' help, these guys were not going to get away with anything. The minute someone put their personal pride on the line, she knew they were trustworthy. She could have ended the interview right then, but as a seasoned pro, she knew to ask a few more questions.

"So, have you ever been approached by someone outside of TemePhelps about bringing in, ah, alternative materials?" she asked.

"No way," he quickly replied.

"Have you ever witnessed anyone inside TemePhelps indicate that they would be bringing in materials other than those you were expecting?" she asked.

"No way," he quickly replied again.

She thumbed through the papers in front of her, jotted some notes on a pad next to her and waited until she thought the appropriate amount of time had passed before declaring the interview over.

"Thank you for your time, Mr. James."

She stood up, shook his hand, and walked to the door with him. Charlie was waiting in the hallway outside. Kat excused herself for a short bathroom break and asked him to wait for her in the conference room. While she was alone, she checked the time. It was after 1:30. That was why her stomach was growling. Now she had to decide whether to take a break for lunch or just plow through for another hour or so and knock off early and maybe get a chance to visit Bernie before dinner. While she was deciding, her phone rang.

"Hey Kat, it's Jimmy. You still in town tomorrow night?"

"Yeah, why?"

"I got these two tickets to a thing at the Kammerly Center."

Kat hesitated. The offer was tempting, since sitting alone in a hotel room could be just plain depressing, and by tomorrow she just might need some company.

"Hmmm, maybe—"

"Great. I'll swing by the hotel and grab you about seven o'clock," he said.

He hung up before she could even ask him what to wear. She was momentarily annoyed, then relieved. There was something nice about someone else just making a decision for you. It had been a while since she had someone to do the give and take with and she missed it more and more.

Now Kat knew she would plow through the rest of the day at TemePhelps, maybe grab a few minutes with Bernie and then relax in a long bath and hit the sack early. She faced another day of grueling inspection, but then had a night out to look forward to. Her excitement was tempered with some apprehension after how Jimmy was the other night. She really didn't want a night of talking about how much these days suck compared to the good old days.

Once back in the room with Charlie, Kat asked whether they could grab something to eat first and he gladly offered to have something sent in. He asked Louise to place the sandwich orders and she disappeared. In the absence of the scribe, neither Charlie nor Kat spoke. Kat looked over reports. Charlie sat, rubbing his eyes.

After a mediocre tuna sandwich and another couple of hours of talking with Charlie, Kat was ready to knock off for the day. She hadn't really uncovered anything that helped her get to the bottom of the MedWatch reports, but she was fairly well convinced that nothing out of the ordinary was happening at this TemePhelps facility. The next part of the puzzle was to step down into the next tier of the supply chain and that meant distributors. Just the thought of it make Kat tired. For every one manufacturer there could be hundreds of distributors, and isolating the one who might be causing a problem was like the proverbial needle in a haystack. She sighed at the thought of how long it might take to isolate the problem, worrying about how many more people might be injured or die while she was investigating. Those were the kinds of thoughts she had to banish from her head, because they would either lead to total despair or sloppy investigating. Neither option would be helpful in tracking down whoever was behind these incidents.

***

Philadelphia was dingy gray in the waning days of winter. Colton was still out of sorts from having to leave his tropical paradise and get back to the States. He rolled out of bed with a plan to get some business out of the way early, attend the Kammerly fundraiser, and then concentrate on preparing for tomorrow night's evening with Cherie and the Wentworths.

But even before he made it to his office, there was trouble. Thanks to Jackie's incompetence, what started out as minor difficulties escalated into the kind of day that might drive him to violence. There were three ways to solve every problem: force, intimidation, or bribery. Today he was going to have to employ all three.

"I'm just gonna meet with the guy myself," he declared.

He watched as beads of sweat rose up on Jackie's upper lip.

"You sure that's a good idea, Boss?" asked Jackie.

Colton ignored the remark. For the third time Jackie had failed to get the Chinese in line, so now he was making excuses, protecting himself from Colton's wrath. He had no choice but to take the Chinese on himself.

"Jackie, tell Reggie we're going to Jersey," barked Colton.

"You and me?" he replied.

"No, me and Reggie. I don't need you there if I'm there. But I wouldn't have had to go if you had done your job right. Right? Another example of why you aren't cut out to run this business," said Colton.

Jackie stood silent, staring off into space.

"Go get Reggie!" Colton yelled.

Jackie sauntered out of the office.

Colton set up his operation with great precision, taking advantage of DeAngelo Sr.'s legitimate trappings. He built his own operation using some of the same connections, but burying them so deep that the feds would never associate his underground operation with USA Distributors. With fists full of cash, he easily found a few inside guys at the manufacturers to lend him a few secrets and soon he was on his way with proprietary formulas and replicas of tablet dies so he could produce the most accurate counterfeits on the market. He approached the Chinese to manufacture for him and that's where he found his biggest headaches. They just didn't understand the culture of business or the nature of a gentleman's agreement. Time and time again he had to set them straight about how business was conducted. They apologized repeatedly before going back to doing exactly what he had just told them not to do. Colton soon realized that apologizing was just something they did to shut him up. The way to move things along in China was with violence. As much as he tried to explain these concepts to Jackie, he never seemed to get it and too often Jackie allowed the Chinese too much leeway.

"You sure you don't want me to come along?" Jackie asked as Colton walked past him on the way to the front door.

Jackie was sweating and pacing. He really wanted the answer to be no.

"Yeah, I want you along. I want you to pull the trigger," he said.

Jackie tried to make his face calm, but Colton could see that how his lip twitched at the corner. He shifted from foot to foot.

"Ah… I, ah… sure Colton, I'll, ah—"

Much as Colton enjoyed the game, he had no intention of taking Jackie with him, nor would he ever put Jackie in charge of enforcement.

"I'm just fuckin' with you, Jackie. Stay here, but take the list from my desk and get everything done. I'll be back in a couple of hours."

Jackie tried to hide it, but Colton saw him heave a sigh of relief. He bit the inside of his lip to keep from laughing.

Colton hit the road with Reggie and made it to the warehouse in about an hour. There was a lot of activity at the far end of the building, with trucks in the docks and workers unloading the trucks, but the rest of the place was pretty quiet. He waited in the car for a minute, scanning the parking area for the Chinese guys. There were a few cars in the lot and he guessed the Chinese owned the black Mercedes with the darkened windows. Since he couldn't see inside, he waited to see in anyone got out of the car. He wanted them in the warehouse before he walked in. After about fifteen more minutes of no activity, he grew impatient, got out of the car and headed up to the loading dock. He motioned for Reggie to stay back at the car and stepped up onto the loading dock just as Lionel, head of warehouse operations, came out.

"Hey, Boss, what brings you here?" he asked, sticking out his hand to shake.

"Checking up on you Lionel. Always checking up on you," Colton replied, clapping Lionel on the back while he shook his hand.

"You want me to get my dad?" Lionel asked.

"Yeah, sure. Tell him I'm here."

Lionel sprinted inside to the warehouse office. Colton liked Rack and his son. They were good workers who knew how to keep their mouths shut. The "no snitchin" culture of the Philadelphia neighborhood where they lived made them similar to the wise guys that came out of the mob neighborhoods of South Philly he worked with in his dealing days. The difference was that Rack and his son were much smarter than most of the South Philly guys. They were also better at relationships with all nationalities of illegals in the area—Hispanic, Russian, Irish, and Nigerian—illegals who worked hard and had a vested interest in not getting deported. They never brought any attention to themselves or Colton's business, just worked hard, took their money and disappeared.

Rack also kept very good records. Perfect in fact. "Ah, now see—sloppy of deed is sloppy of mind," Rack would always say. It wasn't long before Colton trusted him with the cash shipments from the Chinese and stopped being on-site when the money arrived. USA Distributors paid market price to Colton's Chinese plant from whom they purchased raw goods and oral dosage forms. Or so it looked on the books. USA Distributors was actually purchasing substandard raw goods to move into manufacturing, using counterfeit oral dosage forms to blend with what was bought from legitimate sources. And, he was purchasing cash, U.S. dollars, though the invoices reflected pharmaceuticals. Colton kept a portion of the cash to deposit into Swiss accounts and used the rest to distribute.

"Hey, Boss. Good to see you. What brings you to the swamps? Meeting with the Chinese?" asked Rack in his booming voice as he bounded toward Colton.

Colton's hand was completely enveloped by Rack's large mitt. This was a guy who could crush whoever got in his way, a guy who did once crush opponents on the football field before a knee injury ended his hopes and dreams.

"Yeah. They here?" Colton asked.

"Got here a couple of minutes ago. Routine or something up?"

"Supply problems. And following up on the quality issues you brought to me. Any changes better or worse?"

"The last go 'round was better. But I even had to pull about one out of four of those. Got some over here if you wanna look."

Colton followed Rack over to some cardboard barrels, pulled off the lid and opened the heavy plastic liner inside to expose the tablets. Colton stuck his hand in and grabbed a handful of pills and examined them. He could see immediately that they were not pressed nor coated properly. Loose powder flecked off and covered his hand, they were not perfectly shaped, and the colors were not quite perfect. These would never pass off in the legitimate market. They'd have to go to secondary markets either overseas, on the street, or to some government program. Street price might make up for most of the loss, but only for those drugs that had any street value like painkillers. Others, like everyday drugs, would have to be pawned off on Internet pharmacies, or maybe even moved to nursing homes. Colton didn't like being in the street market, this was not the business model he had built.

"Those were some of the worst I've seen," Rack said.

"What are they?" Colton asked.

"Vioxx," Rack replied.

"Not even any street value then," said Colton.

"'Fraid not. Gonna have to go 'net," said Rack shaking his head.

Colton felt his blood boil. He tossed the handful of pills toward the barrel and slapped his hands together to get rid of the loose powder. Rack handed him a baby wipe from a box on a nearby shelf. As he wiped his hands, Colton surveyed the warehouse, thinking as he counted the number of barrels of lousy goods the Chinese had dropped on him. Things had gotten tough since the Heparin mess and the FDA put so much pressure on the Chinese government that his plant had been temporarily shut down. Thanks to some expensive payoffs, his formulas and dies had been moved to another plant, but now he was back to the same kinds of quality issues that plagued his initial production. He had to find out whether these new guys could be made to do a better job or whether he had to scout out yet another new plant.

He hated going to China. Business there was never clean, never easy, the food was rotten, and the whores giggled too much. The first time he went to China, he was excited, thinking he would be conducting meetings like here in the States or over in England where he opened his second plant. But the Chinese had an entirely different set of customs and rules, most of which were painfully slow and aggravating. First, he had to hire an interpreter and then he had to hire a guy to act as his business liaison. By the time he got the business liaison, he had been in China for more than a week eating lousy food and fucking skinny, flat-assed Chinese teenagers. He was becoming more miserable and making it known to Yuan, the liaison, that his patience was wearing thin. In response, Yuan spent a lot of time educating him on Chinese customs and entertaining him, but from what he could see, little time making the right connections for him to conduct his business. It wasn't until he pulled out a gun and stuck it in Yuan's mouth that he finally got a meeting with Mr. Chen, a government official who claimed to have entrée into plants and operators.

Colton trusted Chen as soon as he met him. The guy was fat, a reliable sign that he was someone with money and influence. Mr. Chen claimed to have access to government officials at every level and, soon after Colton paid him a thousand dollars, doors began to open. Mr. Chen got them inside the plant where pharmaceutical raw ingredients were processed for bulk shipment to manufacturing plants around the world. Much as Colton was interested in a source for raw ingredients that he could step on with additives, he also needed an actual oral dose manufacturing facility. He had the dies, he had the source for the ingredients, he had the formulas—what he needed was someplace that would produce the actual tablets. Mr. Chen and another guy assured him that a facility would be found.

But these guys wasted more of Colton's days and probably would have continued to string him along, until he threatened to pull out completely and head over to India. Finally, Mr. Chen set up a series of meetings at government-run plants and even helped work out the logistics to get started. Still, it took an entire year for the first lot to come out of the plant. He flew back to China to give his personal approval and had to control himself as he watched the first lot spill down the shoot and into the barrels. Every single pill was a perfect replica of the real thing. A perfect counterfeit. He could almost smell the money.

Most of the Chinese chemical engineers were young Western-educated Chinese guys, some who graduated from his own alma mater, and all were very, very good at what they did. They knew that the likelihood of the FDA inspecting the facility was tiny; at the current rate, facilities were inspected about once every 13 years. They also knew what the FDA would look for if they ever did get inspected and they were brilliant at faking the lot testing, logs—all the paperwork. He was impressed, though he knew better than to show these guys he was pleased. Instead, he grabbed a few pills, pretended to intensely examine them, then handed them to Mr. Chen with a vague nod. He issued a perfunctory verbal approval and announced that he would be back to inspect again in a few months. Colton's heart raced as he walked away, his face flushed with the knowledge that he had just quadrupled his profits.

"Where are they?" Colton asked Rack.

"There were over there with the warehouse guys, unloading knockoff iPhones for spending money. Let me find 'em for you," said Rack.

Colton paced around the warehouse while he waited for Rack to flush out the Chinese guys. He stepped out onto the loading dock to signal to Reggie to come here with him now, instead of standing by the car. He ran his hand over his hip pocket, feeling the bulge of the switchblade.

Rack returned in another minute, followed by two Chinese guys—one middle aged and another much younger.

They looked like they had stepped straight out of a Quentin Tarantino movie, dressed in a combination of rice racer street wear and thrift store business suits. Colton shook his head, amused. The two approached, stone faced, sporting aviator dark glasses that hid their eyes, walking with a swagger that annoyed Colton.

"You're late," Colton barked.

The men stopped a few feet from him and stood silent. Colton let out a long, exasperated sigh. Reggie put his hand on his pocket and widened his stance and Rack took one step closer to Colton.

"So, tell me about this," Colton demanded as he pointed to the barrels of goods.

The older guy started to yammer on in Chinese while the younger one spoke in English. Colton held up his hand and shook his head.

"English only!" Rack bellowed.

The two guys took a pause, then the older one began to speak English.

"Bad batch," he said and shrugged.

"I can see it's a fucking bad batch! Why'd it happen and what are you going to do about it?!"

Colton heard his voice echo around the warehouse. He clenched his teeth and jutted his chin out and itched to snatch the dark glassed off their faces.

"We fix already," said the older one.

The younger one made a grand gesture out of folding his arms across his chest. Colton took a step closer to the two.

"So, when's the new shipment coming in?" he asked.

"One today," said the older one.

"You'll be here when it arrives and I'll be back to personally inspect," Colton instructed.

"Can't. We got other business in New York," interjected the younger Chinese.

Colton narrowed his eyes and tensed the muscles in his arms. He wanted to smack the kid right then and there.

He never had these kinds of problems in England and if it wasn't that the Chinese worked so damn cheap, he would pull out entirely. The Chinese had no monopoly on guys willing to participate in illegal operations and government officials content to turn their heads for a pocketful of cash.

"Boss says you're back here *today* with the shipment for inspection," said Rack.

The two Chinese men stood silent, stoic, heads cocked. Colton felt the blood pounding at his temples. Now he was going to have to do something memorable to get the correct message across to these guys and he wasn't in the mood to work up a sweat or risk getting blood on his new silk polo. Colton looked at Reggie, then at Rack. Reggie grabbed the young guy while Rack grabbed the older one and held their arms tightly behind their backs. Colton snatched the sunglasses off the faces and flung them across the warehouse. They landed with a "tink" and slid across the bare cement floor. Colton slowly slid a switchblade out of his pocket and flipped open the blade. It made a quiet click as it locked into place. The blade, though not terribly long, was shiny and sharp and felt balanced, natural, in Colton's hand. He took one step closer to the men and surveyed them head to toe, picking lint off of their rumpled jackets and casually tossing it aside, teasing them. He raised the blade slowly toward the young man's face and hovered around for a while, taunting him, threatening to take out an eye, part of a lip, an earlobe maybe, or just inflict a deep cut to the face. He had not yet decided. If these were his own crew, flashing the knife might have been enough, but Colton knew the Chinese learned lessons the hard way. He also knew that even with their modern, capitalist sensibilities, losing face was not just an abstract concept. He knew that culturally it very much mattered to them. A scar on the face would prove that they had lost face in America and make it very difficult for them to continue to work here, make it even more difficult to regain stature among their cohorts in China.

He drew the blade closer to the young man's face and relished the fear in his eyes. Then, with one swift movement, sliced the man's face from the outside corner of his eye, across his cheek and to the tip of his mouth. Blood began to freely flow down his face and soon dripped onto his comical jacket where it soaked in. Colton wanted to stand and savor the blood and what he thought he detected as a tear in the man's eye, but he knew he had to strike the other man immediately, before he had a chance to swallow his fear and become defiant again. The cut to the second man landed with the same accuracy in spite of the fact that the older man flinched.

"Now, tell me what you are going to do today," Colton said calmly, quietly.

In spite of the wounds, neither man spoke and Colton had to wield the weapon again to get them to cooperate. Finally, the older man spoke.

"We will return when the shipment comes in," he said.

"Good, good. I'll be back then too. And we'll all have a look-see together, okay? Then we'll talk about what we do next," he said.

Colton grabbed a wipe from the box on the nearby shelf and methodically cleaned off the blade of his knife. When he was finished, he closed the blade and slid it back into his pocket, balled up the bloody wipe and dropped it on the floor. He motioned to Reggie and Rack and each released the man from their grip. The young man immediately pressed the back of his hand against the wound on his face, checked his soaked hand, then used the sleeve of his jacket to soak up the blood. The older man stood defiant and allowed his wound to bleed all over himself. If Colton didn't understand how dangerous the older man's defiance was, he would have laughed at the sight of him. But he understood and also knew that the man saw that Colton Barnes was not some pretty white boy afraid to dirty his hands.

"Boss said to take off now and make sure you're here with the shipment this afternoon," said Rack.

The two men strolled out of the warehouse and Colton watched as they pulled away in the Mercedes. They may have kept appearances of an attitude but Colton knew he had rattled them. He knew they would be back again but didn't trust that they would have a shipment with them. The Chinese loathed feeling outsmarted, even when it appeared that they were cooperating. They would find a way to get the upper hand. They would return and maybe they would have a shipment, but it would not be a complete shipment and it might not be all the same goods. Still, he would accept it while making his displeasure known and know that the next time his shipment would be quality and complete.

"How much other stuff was bad?" Colton asked Rack.

"Not seeing a lot," Rack replied.

"We have enough supply for how long?" he asked.

"We could go a couple more weeks," Rack replied.

Colton calculated the lead-time from China to warehouse and decided that he could get by for now, but he made a note to call Oliver in the Manchester facility and see whether he could step up production for the short term. The Chinese would have to pay the extra if he had to go that route, just for the trouble they put him through.

"What time you expecting the afternoon trucks?" Colton asked.

"Usually swing in around four-thirty or five o'clock, at the latest," answered Rack.

"Call me if it looks like they'll be in sooner."

Colton motioned to Reggie that it was time to go, and Reggie headed for the Escalade. As he was leaving, Colton stepped over to some warehouse guys who were huddled together around an iPhone they had picked up from the Chinese. When they saw him approach, they quickly hid the item, like children caught with contraband in front of the teacher at school.

"How good is it?" Colton asked.

"Could easily pass as the real thing," said the one guy who held the device behind his back.

Colton held out his hand and motioned for the young guy to hand it over to him, which he did will little hesitation. The other two guys shuffled their feet and looked as though they were about to take off to other parts of the warehouse. Colton took the iPhone from the young guy and turned it over in his hands, memorizing the marks, feeling the weight and dimension, sizing it up to his own genuine iPhone.

"Almost could have fooled me. How much?" he asked.

"Hundred bucks," the young man replied.

"Not bad," Colton said.

He tossed the counterfeit iPhone back to its owner, then left the warehouse and got into the waiting Escalade. He still marveled at how quickly and accurately the Chinese were able to copy just about anything and pondered how huge he could become if he branched out from pharmaceuticals. One day, he thought, one day—but for now the Chinese fucks have to prove that they could get his supply of drugs right.

Chapter 4

Form FDA 3500A, Incident #154:

…Thirty-year-old female developed anemia during second trimester of pregnancy and physician prescribed an iron supplement. Approximately one month later when patient returned, blood panels indicated continued anemia. Additional test results confirmed elevated liver enzymes and limited liver function; patient was counseled to continue iron supplements and schedule consult with specialist. One week later, patient reported nausea, diarrhea, and fatigue and was diagnosed with flu-like symptoms. Symptoms persisted and one week later patient was rushed to the emergency room in premature labor and acute liver failure. Aggressive course of action taken to cease labor without success. Baby was delivered prematurely at 24 weeks. Mother died within 12 hours of delivery. Baby lived additional 48 hours before also expiring.

Initial conclusion was that patient's low iron was the complicating factor in pregnancy, although the subsequent liver failure was unexplained. Patient's iron supplement was tested and found to have been formulated with methanol rather than ethanol…

***

There was thankfully little traffic on the Turnpike as Kat made her way back from the Lancaster County AmPharm facility to West Philly. Her second inspection day was shorter than the first, though more exhausting, partially because her frustration level was rising as her searches turned up nothing.

Yesterday she had gone back to the hotel, exhausted without even stopping to say hello to Bernie. Now she missed the little bugger. There was just enough time for a quick snuggle before she had to be ready for Jimmy. She waited at the frat house door, looking forward to a big slobbering mess of enthusiasm, but instead got only a wag of the tail as Bernie clung to Albe.

"I was afraid of that," she frowned.

"Don't worry about it Mom. How can you compete with a house full of commotion?" asked Albe.

"I know. But still…".

"I'm sure he'll be excited to go home with you in the end." Martha's words held some reassurance, but not much.

"Well, I guess I have time to change now since Bernie doesn't need my company," Kat said. "Is there any place nearby where I can pick up something to wear?"

"That's Martha's department," deferred Albe, stepping back from the door to let Martha onto the porch with Kat.

"What are you looking for?" she asked.

"I got an invitation to this thing at the Kammerly Center tonight and I guess I could wear this…" she motioned to the rumpled suit that currently hung on her frame.

Martha's eyes grew wide and Albe cringed. Kat looked down. She had to agree with their verdict.

"I'll walk you to a couple of places nearby," offered Martha.

Kat was a little uncomfortable at the prospect of shopping for clothing with her son's young girlfriend, but then brightened. It might be the perfect opportunity to get information that she would never get out of Albe. Though she had no signs of it, she always worried that losing his father took a huge toll on Albe, and that somehow led to some secret agonies that her son struggled with and never shared with her.

The two women stopped in a couple of nearby boutiques, but the clothes were too ethnic or too college for Kat and probably not appropriate for something at the Kammerly Center. They ended up at the only store left on the block and that was the GAP. Kat waited until they were inside combing through racks before beginning her questions.

"So, I'm going to be the nosey mother now and ask how long the two of you have been going out, since Albe never tells me these things," Kat said.

"You won't have to drag it out of me. I already expected questions and I told Albe that I would answer them all. We met thirteen months ago at a frat party. It was kind of like we knew from the first meeting that we had a lot in common and wanted to hang out. He's as serious about school as I am, so there's no whining about not having enough time together. We just see each other when we can. But, I can tell you for me, what's between the two of us is serious," she said.

Kat stopped and looked at the girl who continued to pick through the clothing on the racks and hardly flinched at delivering the news of how she felt about Kat's only child. Kat's jumble of emotions, some elated, some sad, churned around in her chest.

"Does Albe feel the same way?" she asked.

"He'd damn well better," Martha replied.

She looked up at Kat and laughed, but Kat didn't know whether to laugh or not.

"It's a joke. Yes, he feels the same way I'm sure. That's why he wanted us to meet," she said.

Kat smiled at the girl and retreated back to the racks for a break from her emotions. She didn't stay silent for long, considering this a rare opportunity and one not to be taken lightly.

"So, how is Albe? I mean, how does he… I worry a lot about him…without his father…"

"He gets sad sometimes," Kat replied. "I'm lucky because I'm close to my dad and I'll just call and talk to him about whatever, just for minute, like if I see something funny, something he'll get a kick out of. And I know that's hard on Albe."

Martha pulled a couple of skirts from the rack and waved them in front of Kat. She stepped back and squinted as if that would help her imagine if either one would work, knowing neither one would, but she wanted to be polite. Martha was astute, she shoved them back onto the rack.

"I still miss him too," Kat admitted.

Martha stopped rifling through the rack and looked directly at Kat.

"It must be hard without either of them with you, huh?" she asked.

Kat felt her eyes well up and abruptly turned her back on Martha and began digging through the rack in front of her. She was embarrassed but relieved to know that Albe found exactly the kind of girl who understood how important it was for him to stay close to his mother.

"How about a black wrap dress?" asked Martha as she yanked the flowing garment off the rack and held it up.

"Looks good." Kat grabbed the dress and practically sprinted to the dressing room.

To her surprise, Martha followed her and waited outside. Kat figured that meant Martha expected to see it when she tried it on, which made her a bit nervous. She had gotten used to shopping alone now and wasn't used to making decisions with an audience. After Jorge's death, she didn't shop at all, but then her friends forced her out of the house one day on an outlet adventure. With only some gentle prodding she ended up with some nice things, but, more importantly, she realized what a favor they had done for her. Still, between extra hours at work and trying to get used to her new life as a widow, shopping didn't grab her attention much. She would buy something only when necessary for work, because outside of the occasional dinner with friends, she had no reason for a lot of clothes.

"So, what's this you're going to?" Martha called from the other side of the dressing room door.

"Oh, an old friend has tickets to some charity thing at the Kammerly Center and asked if I wanted to tag along," she replied.

"Old friend as in old *girl* friend or old *boy* friend?" Martha asked.

Kat shot herself a look in the mirror, amazed at Martha's boldness.

"Boy… but he's an old friend," she quickly added.

"Married?" Martha asked.

"Of course not! Divorced. And just so you know, I would never spend time with a married man. He's just an old *friend*."

She heard Martha hum the kind of humming that has a lot of innuendo attached to it. Kat stopped for a moment trying to decide how she felt about the humming. She could launch into an adamant denial of any interest in Jimmy but that would be insincere. She could reveal that she was interested but she didn't know Martha well enough for that yet. Finally, she slipped on the dress and turned to look at herself in the mirror. The years had certainly taken their toll, but she didn't look bad for a forty something. She looked at least as good as Jimmy did after all these years. The look of herself in the dress replaced her contemplation of Martha's humming.

"So?" she asked as she stepped out of the dressing room and presented herself.

"Very, very nice," said Martha.

"Okay enough for the Kammerly Center?"

"And the divorced 'friend', ah, date," she said.

Martha offered a sly grin and Kat wagged her finger at the girl, but secretly she was pleased. This was the first time she had even let a thought of seeing another man creep into her head and she understood what a turning point it was.

"Maybe you've got time for a haircut?" asked Martha in a small voice.

Kat laughed. "You mean a style?" she said.

Martha quickly nodded.

"There's a place just around the corner. You don't need an appointment," she offered.

After dress shopping, a haircut, and a color, Kat had just enough time to shower and change before Jimmy picked her up. It felt good to want to get dressed up, but it made her a little nervous too. Maybe Jimmy had nothing of the sort in mind and maybe she was overstepping a boundary. She decided to tuck her anticipation carefully away and consider the evening only as an invitation from an old friend who didn't want her hanging out alone in a hotel room.

"So, what's this we're going to?" she asked as she settled into the front seat of Jimmy's car.

"Fundraising event. A lot of the money folks… I have to say, you look great tonight, Kat!"

Kat blushed. She couldn't even look at Jimmy anymore. She tugged at the ends of her hair, fidgeted in her seat, and desperately tried to think of something to say.

"Ah, what were you saying about tonight?" she finally asked to fill the silence.

"Oh, it's a fundraising event. Rich folks in the city are invited to get acquainted with one another while they bid on donated items. You know, the typical charity event these days. The guy dating the woman who organized the event is the son of Joe Barnes, 'Daddy,' the former pro football coach," he explained.

"The guy on NFL Talk?" she asked.

"Same. The son is Colton Barnes. He's one of the largest wholesale drug distributors on the East coast," he said.

"Ah, competitor of yours," she said.

"Right. Gotta stay in contact with these guys, you know, in case they want to buy us out some day," said Jimmy.

Now Kat did look at Jimmy, who was keeping his eyes on the road.

"You selling?" she asked.

"No, but I don't want to work forever either." He glanced in her direction, but she quickly turned her head away.

Kat filed the information in the back of her head. Tonight was about having fun with an old friend, not FDA business.

There was a line to get into the Kammerly Center and Kat and Jimmy waited outside on Broad Street for about fifteen minutes before they could get inside. The lobby was teeming with people, well-dressed people, and Kat felt a bit embarrassed at her simple GAP dress, in spite of Jimmy's gushing compliment. At least she let Martha talk her into a large cuff bracelet, some strands of chains and beads, a red clutch and, thankfully, a new hairstyle and color.

At one end of the lobby was a stage where a jazz combo played. Four bars were set up at various locations around the room and numerous white-gloved attendants circulated the room with trays of finger food. Jimmy led Kat over to one of the bars where they each got a drink—him a beer, her a glass of champagne. They made their way over to the table with the auction items.

"What should I bid on?" he asked.

"How much you got to spend?" she replied.

"If it's charity, I've got double the budget, so it's about $5,000," he said.

Kat was a little taken aback. Her salary had downscaled when she left the pharmacy profession to work for the FDA. There was the money from the Klein civil case but most of that went to pay off her mortgage and Albe's tuition at Penn. She tucked the rest into her retirement account.

Kat perused the listings of items and picked out a couple of things that sounded interesting and pointed them out to Jimmy. He marked them on his sheet and then the two of them made their way over to a quieter spot where they could talk and survey the room.

"So who's here that I might be interested in?" she asked.

"You recognize Daddy Barnes. That's Colton to his left and I guess the girl on his arm is Cherie Fulton, the girlfriend and the charity event organizer I was telling you about," he replied.

Barnes, a surprisingly plain and short man compared to his father, was dressed in a classic black tuxedo. Cherie, the petite, raven-haired beauty, wore a burgundy-beaded gown that clung to her curvy figure.

"They certainly look like they're some of the beautiful people," Kat remarked.

"Beautiful and well connected. Bitsy Kammerly is next to Cherie. On the other side of Daddy are Langford Wentworth— old money lawyer—and his wife Patricia. The rest of the crowd around him are probably prominent lawyers, judges and politicians," said Jimmy.

"Who're the thugs?" Kat asked, referring to the burly looking guys that flanked the younger Colton.

"Former players for coach?" speculated Jimmy.

Maybe, but Kat thought had her doubts. She watched them survey the crowd, periodically checking in with each other with nods and signals and the occasional comment into their sleeve. They looked more like bodyguards and wondered why a guy like Colton needed bodyguards. Kat studied the group of people, particularly those who swarmed around Colton, if only because he seemed awfully young to be so connected and so successful. Then again, when you have the help of a famous and beloved father, many more doors opened easier and wider. Kat noticed that father and son were none too keen on talking with one another and even caught some moments when Daddy must have thrown a barb at Colton, who kept a stern face while Daddy and those around him laughed heartily.

Cherie excused herself from the group and made her way to the stage with the help of Colton, who held onto her elbow as she scaled the steps in her towering heels. When the jazz combo spotted her, they wound down on the number they were playing and turned the microphone over to her.

"Good evening ladies and gentlemen and thank you all so much for joining us this evening. Welcome to the annual charity auction to benefit the magnificent Kammerly center. Thanks to Ralph and Bitsy Kammerly, the center has become the cultural apex of Philadelphia and the largest gem here on the Avenue of the Arts. We had another spectacular year of performances from the Philadelphia Orchestra, all the guests of the ProBank Jazz series and a number of other headliners who help insure that the music scene in the city of Philadelphia continues to thrive. But as you know, we cannot do this alone and that's where we turn to you for help. All proceeds from this evening's auction will benefit the center, so please be generous. Now, I'd like to introduce Bitsy Kammerly, who will say a few words."

An ethereal Bitsy dressed in a stunning white gown with gold trim, approached the microphone and said a few words to open the auction. A parade of auction item donors joined Cherie and the auctioneer as their item was bid on. And though it was interesting to see what caught people's fancy, it was even more interesting to witness the results of internal politicking among Philadelphia's elite. The "old" money huddled on one side of the lobby and the nouveau riche stayed to themselves on the other side. Kat remembered the old money names—prominent Philadelphian names, the kinds of names that graced buildings or hospital wings or companies still in operation. But she easily recognized the new names of sports stars, investment moguls, actors, and authors. Interestingly, Daddy Barnes and his son, Colton, seemed to be the ones to bridge the gap between the two groups. They were quite the operators, shaking hands, making people laugh, and generally ingratiating themselves with the power elite.

"That's the end of that," said Jimmy.

"What?" Kat asked.

She had been so busy watching the people that she was paying no attention to the auction itself.

"Just lost the tickets to see the Eagles with Daddy Barnes," he said.

"Oh, well, isn't the weekend getaway still up for auction?" she asked hopefully.

Jimmy nodded vaguely and went back to paying attention to the auction while Kat continued to watch the room. At one point, she saw an exchange between Colton and his father. Colton stormed away and slammed down a couple of drinks at the bar before returning.

"So who did you say the Wentworth guy was?" she asked.

"Langford Wentworth. You remember Albert Wentworth from the Wilson murder trial? The attorney for the trial of the century?" Jimmy asked.

"That was about the basketball star accused of murdering his wife and mother, right?"

"The case made the already famous Wentworth even more famous and multiple millions in the aftermath. His son, Langford, was Colton's roommate at Penn," Jimmy replied.

Kat briefly thought of what an unlikely combination that must have been.

"It's pretty common knowledge, though, that Daddy over there doesn't much like his own kid because he turned out to be pretty pathetic at football," Jimmy added.

"You know him?".

"I've had some dealings with the kid, just in passing. Professional. Seemed okay to me," he said.

The auction drew to a close and Jimmy hadn't been able to get so much as one item that was in his budget. It seemed to bother him, although she couldn't quite figure out why. She decided to get his mind off of the auction.

"You hungry?" she asked.

"Yeah. Let's get out of here and grab some dinner." He turned back to her, focusing for her for the first time all night, smiled and took her arm.

They began to make their way to the doors but the crowd thickened and they were not able to move until it began to thin out. Meanwhile, Daddy Barnes, Colton, and the Wentworths were walking out with the crowd and came closer to where Jimmy and Kat were waiting. Kat tried to be nonchalant with her gaze and not stare, but something about them was just mesmerizing, charismatic. As they got closer, the burly guys that Kat spotted earlier created a kind of buffer zone between them and the rest of the exiting public. Still, Kat was close enough to overhear some of what Daddy Barnes was saying to Langford.

"Maybe that knucklehead son of mine will finally ask that girl to marry him, although I don't know why she would! See, Langford, you're the kind of guy who successfully followed in his father's footsteps. That kid of mine doesn't know a shotgun formation from a blitz!"

"Well, I wish I could say that he was the academic type instead. But that's not the case either," Wentworth replied.

"Sometimes I think his mother must have fucked the mailman," said Daddy.

"We could always have a paternity test done, huh, Daddy Joe?" joked Wentworth.

"You hear that," he announced to the crowd. "We're gonna figure out why you're a loser!"

Kat watched Colton's face as he walked behind the two of them. His jaw pulsed as he clenched his teeth and his eyes flashed the anger bubbling inside of him. Kat felt a twinge inside, both at the cruelty of the conversation and how a frightening fury seemed to emanate from Colton's silence. She studied him closely, and as she did, he looked up and caught her eye. She quickly looked away, embarrassed. But catching her eye must have led his gaze to Jimmy and Colton stopped walking and approached him.

"Jimmy Kirk," he stuck out his hand to Jimmy, smiling like the charmer he was.

"Colton, hey, good to see you," said Jimmy, taking his hand.

"Glad you could make it."

"Yeah, me too. Seems like the night went well."

"Very well. Very well. Cherie did another great job."

Kat was trying to look like she wasn't listening to the conversation and that she wasn't associated with Jimmy. She hoped Jimmy would not feel like he had to introduce her.

"Great job. Some great items to bid on," Jimmy continued.

"What'd you get?"

Kat noticed Colton scanning the room

"Ah, couple of things. Laid out some serious cash for you… didn't manage to get that Eagles game with your dad though. That would have been a treat," said Jimmy.

"I'll invite you up to the luxury box sometime when he's there," Colton offered.

Kat tried not to watch as Jimmy practically leapt with excitement at Colton's offer.

"So, how's business? You surviving these days? Last I heard you guys has some troubles over there," Colton said.

Jimmy laughed and shook his head.

"Nah. Must have been someone else. You know, we've got the same issues. The Cantor business with the Heparin. Same as everybody else."

"Crazy huh?" Colton replied.

Kat kept her eyes on the passing crowd as Jimmy and Colton chatted, but she could feel Colton's eyes on her. She thought about striking up a conversation with the guy next to her just to make it look like she was with him. It was hard to resist the temptation to stare at Colton. There was something about him that was both dangerous and sad. From a distance, he seemed like an imposing figure, like his father, but up close, his fidgety insecurities were clearly evident and his thinning hair made him look older. She wondered what about him made him appealing to someone like Cherie, other than his money.

"Listen, good to see you. Oh, I may want to talk to you about another thing soon. Can I call you?" Colton shook Jimmy's hand again.

"Sure. Look forward to it,"

With that, one of the burly guys standing with Daddy Barnes and the others waved to Colton to join them. Colton made his way through the crowd to meet up with his father and the others.

Her gut told her that Colton Barnes was someone she needed to know more about.

She pretended to speak to someone off in the distance until she was sure that Barnes and the others had gotten out the door.

"Sorry I didn't introduce you, but—" Jimmy began.

"No, no. Thank you for not introducing me. With all the stuff that's going down now, it's better that I don't get to know any —"Kat clamped her mouth shut, realizing that she was spending the evening with a company owner she probably shouldn't be spending time with.

"What stuff?" he asked.

"Colton wants to talk with you about a thing, huh?" Kat asked, changing the subject.

"Don't know what that's about," he said.

"Hmmm. Why'd you lie to him about the size of your bid?" she asked.

Jimmy laughed, but Kat could see that he was hiding something. Was there a relationship between Jimmy and Colton Barnes that Jimmy was obviously reluctant to share?

"So, you up for dinner, more drinks or…" Jimmy asked.

Kat filed her suspicion away for the future as they finally made their way out of the Kammerly Center and onto Broad Street..

Kat had already had more than a couple of drinks and enjoyed enough of the delicious snacks that she honestly didn't feel hungry. Then too, she was feeling exhausted from thinking too much in one day and even though she would have loved to have just gone to bed, she still had reports to go over and another inspection at AmPharm to get ready for tomorrow. Of course all of that was a convenient excuse for the peril of continuing to have such a good time with Jimmy.

"I hate to be a killjoy, but I'm not really hungry and I have work to do before I turn in, so I think I'd better get back to the hotel," Kat said.

Jimmy heaved a sigh, but politely obliged and began walking her to the parking garage. As they rounded the corner, a cold wind assaulted them, which sent a shiver through Kat. Jimmy responded by putting his arm around her. She was startled at first, not sure she was interpreting the real meaning of his gesture. It had been more than twenty years since she had dated anyone, more years than anyone could be expected to remember all the nuances of being with someone of the opposite sex that your weren't married to.

Suddenly, as they got near the driveway to the parking garage, Jimmy stopped walking. He gently pushed her against the wall, laying his lips on hers in a passionate kiss. Kat was completely surprised and for a moment thought to push him away, but the feeling of kissing a man after so many years felt too good to pass up and she responded to him. She was startled at how much she enjoyed the taste and feel of him and even allowed herself to think about bringing him back to the hotel with her. But, she banished those thoughts almost as quickly as they entered her mind. He pulled his lips away from hers and spoke.

"Kat, I realized how much I missed you all these years," he said.

It felt good to hear him say that, but she was fairly sure that he was exaggerating. The two of them had been good buddies in school and after, but only romantic teasing passed between them, and one kiss, maybe two, with a lot of flirting but nothing more. Still, she was an adult, one who had not had sex in over five long years and she wondered what the harm would be in seizing on an opportunity for pleasure, especially since she knew the guy was not some kind of crazy.

"Jimmy—"

"Let's go back to the hotel," he whispered to her as he lightly kissed her neck.

It felt so good to have him pressed against her as she inhaled the musty, sweaty man smell of him. In spite of the nagging thought that she had no business doing this with him, she let him take her by the hand and lead her to the car. He opened the door and helped her inside, pausing to kiss her one more time before he closed the door. When he got in the driver's side, he leaned over and kissed her again, this time more sweetly, brushing his hand against the side of her breast and pulling away with a half-smile.

On the ride to the hotel, Kat's nerves and insecurities flooded over her, with worries about her body, the feelings of inadequacy and then, the biggest fear of all, getting pregnant at her age. Too many years had passed where she didn't have to think about that danger, either because she was on the Pill or because there was no Jorge. Now, she felt foolish and had no idea how to broach the subject with Jimmy. Though the possibilities were not great that she could get pregnant, they were still there. She would use them as her excuse to slow this down.

As he pulled up to the hotel, he began to turn into the parking garage.

"Ah, I've got a really busy day tomorrow..."

Jimmy ignored her and pulled into the garage and parked anyway. Without a word, he exited the car and circled around and opened her door. Kat tried to will herself to tell him that he could not come upstairs with her but no words came out of her mouth. Once outside the car, he took her hand in his and led her into the building, then into the elevator to her floor. In her mind she ran over all the reason why she should not be doing this and yet she continued down the hallway to her room without registering any kind of protest, without saying a single word. Somehow she convinced herself that not doing or saying anything to stop where she was heading was different than choosing to continue, almost as though she found it necessary to give herself an alibi to use later. When they arrived at the room, she unlocked the door and entered, then turned, hesitated for only a moment, then held the door open for Jimmy.

***

"Where to now, Boss?" asked Reggie.

Colton checked the dashboard clock and saw he had a few hours to kill before the Chinese came back with the late shipment. *If* the Chinese came back. He debated whether to go back to the office and check on Jackie and the errand list or take off for a few hours. Without doubt, Jackie and the errands would irritate him, often just being around Jackie irritated him. He decided he had enough to deal with today, and deserved some down time before got back to his confrontation with the Chinese.

"How's 'bout a steak and a couple of hands of blackjack?" he asked.

"Hell, yeah," Reggie quickly replied.

Reggie maneuvered them onto the Atlantic City Expressway. Colton called Melinda, the concierge at the Borgata, and put in his reservation for a table at Bobby Flay Steak and a "companion" to meet him there in forty-five minutes. He could tell by Reggie's face that he was disappointed at not being invited to share lunch.

Colton slid five $100 bills out of his pocket and stuffed them between Reggie's hand and the steering wheel.

"Here's for you to have your own fun," he said.

Reggie looked at the bills, grinned and sped up.

A tall, blonde beauty waited for Colton just outside of Bobby Flay Steak, probably the best looking girl Melinda had ever booked for him. He would arrange for an extra tip for Melinda if the girl turned out to be both good company at lunch and a champ in bed.

"I'll bet this handsome man is Mr. Barnes," she said as she held out her perfectly manicured hand for him to shake. She was dressed in a beautifully tailored, white linen sleeveless dress that clung to her curves as though it had been especially made for her.

"You have a good eye," he said as he grasped her hand and gently pulled her toward him so he could kiss her cheek.

He took in her smell and recognized her perfume as Hermes, the same as Cherie. He wondered whether that was accidental or whether Melinda arranged for that special detail too. Female pimps were always the best, so much better at providing what the customer wanted rather than some version of their own personal tastes. And they paid attention to details.

"I'm Kristin," she said as he stepped back from kissing her.

"I hope you like steak," he said, gesturing for her to enter the restaurant before him.

"My favorite," she replied.

They were immediately ushered to their table in the partially filled restaurant. The seating was more open than Colton would have liked, with tables through the middle and only a few cozy booths along one side of the room. Colton didn't want to risk being seen with a woman other than Cherie but he didn't want his style cramped by pretending his lunch with Kristin was strictly business. He scanned the room, and then convinced himself that the danger of being seen by anyone he knew at a restaurant a hundred miles from home on a weekday afternoon was minimal. Still, he insisted on one of the booths and sat with his back to the door.

The two shared light conversation of typical lies about names and business while they enjoyed their drinks and waited for their entrees. Colton felt that Kristin was taken by him, that he was more than just another one of her "dates." In spite of his physical shortcomings, he still moved with the Barnes swagger, and for all of his insecurities, he knew down to his very core that he was a brilliant businessman, on par with Stephen Jobs or Bill Gates. His confidence drew women to him.

"How's the steak?" he asked.

"Delicious," Kristin replied, twirling her fork seductively as she speared a piece of meat and brought it to her mouth.

"Not too spicy?" he inquired.

"Perfect," she purred.

He liked her even more that she ordered the spicy steak, imagining that she preferred other things spicy too. Many men would have skipped the meal and gone right upstairs for the sex but Colton was more aroused by playing out the fantasy of the affair. There was a time he worried that there was something wrong with him that he could not fuck a woman immediately after meeting her. He even went so far as to order a barrage of blood tests to make sure he had no lack of testosterone. As he became more successful, his confidence grew and he no longer compared himself to other men. He also learned from the legions of men in St. Bart's. He saw how they wooed their women, respected them, and yet seemed to adore them. These were hard men, men who had done the unimaginable, yet they were not afraid to be soft and kind to the women with them, even the ones for whom they paid. The mark of true sophistication was to treat your whores as though they were women with whom a relationship mattered.

"Finished?" he asked once their plates were empty.

She smiled at him and rose from her seat. As they exited the restaurant, she brushed her hand against his, a gesture of gentle enticement that thrilled him and sent a twinge to his cock. She followed him to the front desk and stood close beside him as he checked in, gently running her nails up and down his back as he signed for the two of them. Once in the elevator, she leaned into him and allowed him to feel the entire length of her body as it rested against his. Then she kissed him lightly on the mouth, barely touching his lips, teasing him, preparing him. She didn't have to work that hard but he admired her for it.

Their fifteenth floor suite in the Borgata had floor to ceiling windows with an expansive view of the Atlantic City coastline in either direction. From his first glimpse, he envisioned Kristin up against the window where he could feel himself inside of her while he soaked up the panorama. He turned to see her watching him at the window and raised her eyebrows seductively. He smiled.

She removed her dress while keeping her gaze on him and revealed the fine French silk lingerie she wore underneath, revealing yet tasteful, clearly a notch above the trashy, cheap stuff other girls wore. He waited for her to come to him and stood still while she skillfully removed his clothing and respectfully laid it on the couch so it would not wrinkle. He enjoyed many minutes of her sexual virtuosity before he led her over to the window and began acting out his fantasy. She complied completely, and with every thrust inside of her, he took in both the feel of her, the smell of her, and the thought that they were being gazed upon with envy from the mere creatures on the ground below. He finished, then moved away from her and headed to the bedroom to retrieve a robe to wrap around himself. Colton never liked the feeling of walking around naked after sex. His flaccid penis dripping with his cum and her wetness always depressed him.

"Drink?" he asked as he returned in the robe.

She shook her head. "Mind if I take a quick shower?"

Colton gestured to the bathroom, and then walked over to the bar to make himself a drink. She was quick in the shower. Colton had barely taken two sips of his drink before she returned to the room. She was still topless, wearing only remnants of her lingerie on the bottom. He liked the look of her, now that he could take more time to study her, and thought perhaps he might take a go at her one more time.

"How about that drink?" he asked.

"Just some water, if that's okay," she answered politely.

He opened a bottle of ice-cold water and poured it into a glass for her, and then refreshed his Scotch. She retrieved her glass of water and as she did, she brushed against him seductively. As he studied her sweet swinging ass walking away from him, he pondered whether he had time or energy for another go 'round. He was tempted, very tempted, but too unsure that he could go again so soon and unwilling to take the chance.

"I'm going to take a quick shower. Then I have to get going," he said after glancing at his watch.

"Would you like some company?" she asked.

"I would, but I can't be late," he said, excusing himself from the pressure of performing again.

She took a long draw of her water, then set the glass down and dressed herself, aware that he watched her from the next room, tailoring all of her movements to his watchful eyes. Now he knew that he would ask for her again. He would make sure to tip Melinda extra for her fabulous find. This afternoon encounter would serve him well when he was with Cherie tonight and he was glad he resisted the temptation to exhaust himself on Kristin again.

She kissed him lightly before she left and he brushed some stands of her hair away from her face with his fingers. Once she was gone, he showered, dressed, and called Reggie to meet him downstairs.

"How'd you do?" he asked Reggie as he approached.

"Down about a hundred," he replied.

"Not bad," said Colton.

"You?" Reggie asked.

"No gambling today. I'm going to grab a gift for Cherie. Then we can get going." Colton never gambled; he preferred to use his money on sure bets, bets he could control.

He entered the Balenciaga shop at the Borgata. Cherie had been searching for a pair of their jeans last week but grew frustrated with the shop in Rittenhouse Square, which didn't have her size, and seemed less than cooperative to place an order and obtain them for her. If Colton had been there with her, he would have made sure the shop found the jeans, but Cherie was never the type to toss a fit in a shop. She fumed about the experience later with Colton and he offered to straighten the shop out but she refused. He paid a few of Reggie's acquaintances to visit the place anyway and lift about a thousand dollars' worth of merchandise and deliver the message that there were economic consequences to being uncooperative with important customers.

"May I help you, sir?" the middle aged woman asked.

"I'm looking for a certain pair of jeans."

The woman snapped to immediately and led him over to a rack with hanger after hanger of jeans. She pulled out pair after pair until Colton finally recognized the one Cherie had described.

"What size?"

"Ah…" Colton hesitated.

"I'll call Betsy," Reggie offered immediately.

"While your friend is checking on size, is there anything else I might interest you in? A top perhaps?"

Colton surveyed the tops hanging above the jeans and began to get interested until he realized that they seemed to be some kind of shrunken kimono, which reminded him of China. That put him off entirely. He must have winced because the saleswoman quickly steered him into another section.

"Four," said Reggie once he had finished on the phone with Betsy.

"If you would like to continue looking, I will pull that pair of Balenciaga's for you and have them ready behind the counter."

Colton scanned the shop in search of an additional item for Cherie but soon decided that the jeans were enough. Cherie was touchy about clothing gifts and usually preferred to pick them out for herself unless there was a specific item she wanted. Tonight was an important night and he didn't want any complications. Langford and Patricia were coming for dinner and it was imperative that both he and Cherie were in the best of moods to impress the Wentworths. Then it occurred to him that if he also brought a pair of jeans for Patricia, he might have an ace in the hole, especially if it turned out that Patricia was a size larger than Cherie.

"Ask Betsy for Patricia's size," he said to Reggie.

Reggie dutifully called and found out Patricia's size. Colton walked over to the counter where the saleswoman stood and asked for another pair of Balenciaga's, size six. He could hardly contain his smugness. Now his evening with the Wentworths was set. Colton and Reggie exited the shop and headed through the casino and out to the parking garage, but as they reached the door, Colton stopped dead in his tracks and stared across the casino. At the $20 blackjack tables, he spotted Jackie Sr. surrounded by a couple of women and a line of empty glasses that betrayed how long he had been there. Colton contained his anger for the time being and prepared to head across the room and confront Jackie.

"Over there," he said to Reggie, nodding toward the table where Jackie sat.

Reggie whistled through his teeth. "You want me to get him, or you want to?" he asked.

Colton pondered a strategy for a moment, and then decided it would be unseemly for him to approach Jackie Sr. directly. He would wait on the other side of the casino for Reggie to drag Jackie over. He watched as Jackie Sr. whirled around and spotted Colton, a look of panic on his face. He grabbed his chips and headed to the cashier, but Reggie maneuvered him over to where Colton stood instead.

"Pretty good day, huh?" Colton asked.

"Less than half are winnings," Jackie Sr. offered hastily.

"So you won't mind turning over half then," Colton replied.

"Ah, see, I got this guy and—" Jackie Sr. was breathing heavily and was sweating all over the chips in his hands.

"Reggie, how many conversations have we had with this guy about coming to the casinos?" Colton asked.

"Too many," Reggie replied.

"Right. Big Jackie, I just don't understand why you don't learn anything. Isn't this how I got your business in the first place?" Colton asked.

"It's different now."

"One thing I've learned about people is that, in spite of what they say, they just don't change. So, I need you to hand over half and get home now. Otherwise, I'm going to have to put Jackie Jr. on you again and you know how much you hated that, huh?"

Jackie Sr. reluctantly handed over half the chips he clutched to Colton who tried not to react to the feel of the sweaty chips. He watched as Reggie escorted Big Jackie to the cashier where Big Jackie cashed out his chips and pocketed the money. Then Reggie escorted Big Jackie out of the building with orders to make sure he got into his car and headed out of Atlantic City. Colton watched, with a twinge of sadness, the guy who scared him silly when he was a kid, a big, guy, well-connected, successful, blustery guy who was like a real father to him.

Colton was surprised when Jackie Jr. first came to him and confided about his father's gambling problem. Jackie Sr. was the type of guy who was always on top of the world and he could hardly get over seeing him as the loser he had become. He pissed away his life's work at the casinos! How could he have been such a sucker? It didn't take Colton long to realize that Jackie Sr.'s failing could become his opportunity.

He'd already been working in a legitimate lab with some other Penn biochemistry grads, working on assays and compound formulations, but his real bread-and-butter was his expanding street drug business. By the time Colton had graduated from high school he had a thriving street drug business in Philly, but his business really took off when he hit the University of Pennsylvania students and their suburban friends with pockets stuffed full of money. Colton soon realized that he was very, very good at dealing. What he realized later was that dealing brought him all the satisfaction he was missing everywhere else in his life. As the years went on, he began to worry about how long he could continue his enterprise without getting caught. He'd made a lot of friends in law enforcement but understood how tenuous those relationships were. He was always one ambitious district attorney away from losing everything. He foundered around trying to find the perfect substitute for his street business, some other enterprise where he could find as much success and fulfillment. There was nothing. As he was sliding into a funk realizing that his better days might be behind him, Jackie Sr. landed on his doorstep.

Big Jackie accidentally presented him with the perfect solution. It didn't take much to much more than some scary casino thugs to convince Big Jackie to accept Colton's deal: in exchange for baling him out of debt, Colton would take an 80 percent share of USA Distributors. Big Jackie would be well-compensated, taken care of for life, but was never to ask about the business or set foot in a casino again. Jackie Jr. would remain on and run the legitimate side of the business, while Colton had a legitimate front for his continuing illegal operations. The more he learned about the drug wholesaler trade, the more Colton realized that he could get out of the street drug business and make money in the counterfeit business, with little or no risk. He increased his profit margin by using cheaper ingredients and mixing counterfeits with legitimate prescription drugs, all in plain sight.

Colton's chemistry background served him well, as did his connections with Penn grads and pharmacists around the region, none of whom knew or suspected that they were helping him create a less than legitimate enterprise. They trusted him because he was one of their own and they always helped one of their own. Soon he had the formulas in his hands to recreate many of the best selling drugs on the market, and armed with that, he went looking for offshore manufacturers. He approached the Brits first, then the Chinese. He even consulted Langford on business advice and Langford gladly hooked him up with a reputable accounting firm. Colton used them for his legitimate books. Hugh did his other set. He was careful not to expand too quickly, or to move more merchandise than could reasonably be supported with the legitimate books. He was a patient man when he had to be. To build an enterprise that would support him forever required a great deal of patience.

Colton took one last look at Big Jackie and then walked over to the cashier and collected his money from the stack of Big Jackie's chips and shoved it into his pocket. He pulled out a hundred for Reggie and another hundred for Melinda, and then made his way out of the casino and over to the hotel where he spotted her on the phone behind the desk. Her face lit up when she spotted him and he couldn't help but feel a warmth toward her, this woman who took care of him so well with perfect companions.

"I trust your afternoon was satisfactory?" she asked as he approached.

"Much more," he replied.

As he leaned forward to kiss her on each cheek, he slipped the money into her jacket pocket and patted it so she would realize his gesture. She stepped back and smiled broadly at him.

"Will you be returning soon?" she asked.

"I never know but you'll be the first to hear from me when I do," he replied.

"I look forward to it," she said.

He thanked her again and asked her to convey his gratitude and pleasure to her friend. She promised to comply. His business done, he headed back to the casino to find Reggie.

"I made sure he got into his car and followed him to the expressway," Reggie said.

Colton nodded then handed Reggie a $100 bill. "That's for your trouble."

"Thanks, Boss."

Colton gestured and Reggie obliged by walking out to the parking lot to bring the Escalade around to head back to the warehouse.

The Chinese were already there when they pulled into the parking lot, a good sign that they were beginning to understand that they needed to treat him with more respect. He let Reggie exit the car first and check out the Chinese guys' Mercedes, just to make sure there was no hint of an ambush. The car was empty, so Reggie climbed up the loading dock and walked into the warehouse to find the two. A couple of minutes later, Reggie called Colton on the cell and reassured him that the Chinese were inside, politely waiting for him. Colton walked up to the loading dock just as a tractor-trailer pulled around the corner and into a delivery bay.

Reggie and Rack stood next to the two Chinese guys when Colton approached. He had to bite the inside of his lip to keep from smiling at the sight of the two with bandages haphazardly taped to their faces.

"It's here now," said the younger Chinese man.

The driver positioned his rig perfectly in the loading bay then cut off the engine. He walked around to the back of the rig, unlocked the doors, pulled them open and then stepped aside. The trailer was stacked with 55-gallon size fiber barrels lined with plastic, each containing 400 pounds of pills. Next to them, a series of cardboard boxes marked "Scott Paper Company" filled the remaining space. The warehouse crew began to offload the first line of barrels and move them into the warehouse before Colton stopped them.

"Hang on. I want to check contents first. We're not going to waste time unloading if I don't like what I find," he said.

The warehouse workers immediately stopped what they were doing and waited. Colton pulled the lid off of the first barrel and untwisted the plastic liner to inspect the pills inside. Unlike the previous shipments, there was no powder residue on the plastic liner and the pills appeared to be in pristine condition, with correct color, little breakage, crisp shapes. Altogether a much better product. Colton was fairly sure these were legitimate, which meant they probably high jacked a delivery truck somewhere. No matter, they could peddle their sub-standard junk to someone else. What mattered was that he had sent a clear message that he was no sucker and that they either played fair with him or there would be a price to pay.

Colton made a spectacle out of inspecting the pills, pretending that he had more testing secrets than necessary or reasonable, but it was an act that he felt was important to show the Chinese how knowledgeable he was. He ran his fingers through the pills and watched them drop down again, as if that action showed him something about quality. Then, he extracted one pill from deep inside, held it up to his eye and examined it, ran it around between his finger and thumb and finally tasted it. He took a test tube out of his pocket, dropped the pill inside and added a couple of drops of clear liquid from another bottle he had in his pocket. Then he put the stopper securely in the tube, shook the contents hard, and waited. He eyed the Chinese as he pretended to wait for a reaction between the pill and the liquid he put inside. Their faces were expressionless. Finally, he examined the contents of the test tube and declared the shipment acceptable.

When all the barrels were offloaded, he motioned to Rack to have his guys unload the Scott Paper boxes. Two warehouse workers rode over on forklifts, removed the boxes and deposited them in a separate area of the warehouse behind heavy, steel doors with multiple locks. Later, after all the other workers had left, Rack would open each Scott paper box and count the contents, making sure that the amount of cash inside matched what the Chinese were supposed to bring in with the shipment.

Colton watched until everything was out of the tractor-trailer and safe in the warehouse. He knew it was important to show the Chinese how closely he scrutinized his shipments, how they would never be clever enough to outsmart him. He shook hands with Rack, and then left the warehouse without another word

The ride home was uneventful and Colton spent most of the time feeling exhilarated by his victory with the Chinese. This was a turning point in their relationship; from now on he would get only the best quality goods, the best service. From now on, he would get exactly what he was supposed to be getting. The sub-standard stuff would be dumped on someone who didn't have the courage to take on the Chinese.

When he finally got back to the condo, Colton heard Cherie playing the Baldwin from outside the door, meaning she would be relaxed and cheerful this evening. He was quiet as he entered and made his way over to the couch to enjoy the music and the sight of her playing it. She wore clingy black pants and a white tank top that showed off her toned arms. Her hands glided across the keys, expertly, beautifully. Her talent was one of reasons he had bought this condo in the shadow of the Kammerly Center; he would have preferred to settle closer to Rittenhouse Square where the Langfords were, in the most prestigious part of town. But, her enthusiasm for the arts was infectious and useful. Her background helped her become a powerhouse fundraiser for The Kammerly Center and a personal acquaintance of Ralph Kammerly's wife, Bitsy.

Cherie once wanted a career as a performer, but as the years after music school ticked by, she changed her emphasis from performing to a supporter of the arts. Colton met her at one of the fundraisers that Langford and Patricia dragged him to a few years ago. He was immediately struck by her confidence and beauty, and, of course, her connections. He got her number that night and asked her out the following weekend. After only a few dates, he was impressed at how she understood how to remain strong and accomplished in public but soft and accommodating when they were alone, a quality so often lacking in other women her age.

"I'm sorry. I didn't hear you come in," she said as she suddenly stopped playing.

"I was enjoying it," he replied.

She smiled weakly and made a face. She was always too self-critical, a vestige of her conservatory days.

"The caterer should be here soon," she said, rising from the piano bench and starting toward the kitchen.

"I brought you something," he said.

He waited for her to come to him, leaving the bag with the Balenciaga jeans at his feet. She came to him and kissed him lightly on the mouth, then sat down beside him first, then reached into the bag and removed the jeans. A huge smile crossed her face. She leaned over and kissed him again.

"How did you find them?" she asked.

"I was at the Borgata today, in the Balenciaga shop," he said.

"Did you go all the way down there for me?" she asked.

"Of course," Colton lied. "And, I thought Patricia might like a pair too."

Cherie pulled the second pair of jeans out of the bag.

"That's very nice of you," she replied and gave him a long kiss.

He savored her soft lips, enjoyed the smell and feel of her before she leaned back and examined her jeans again.

"What's the dress for tonight?" she asked.

"Though I would love to see you in those, I think maybe not jeans this evening," he replied.

Before she could react, the doorbell rang and she excused herself to answer it. Colton glanced at his watch. The caterer arrived exactly on time and began to set up in the kitchen, while his assistant set up the dining room. Colton watched for a minute, thinking about pouring himself a drink, but all the activity annoyed him. He retreated to the bedroom to get ready for the evening while Cherie supervised. As he was changing into a clean shirt, Cherie entered the bedroom and went straight for the shower.

Colton was relaxing by checking his stock portfolio when Cherie joined him in the study, dressed in a tasteful black dress that clung to her curves and reminded him of Kristin from this afternoon. He was immediately aroused and checked his watch to decide whether he had time before the Wentworths arrived. Cherie must have guessed what went through his mind because she hiked up her dress and climbed onto his lap, straddling her legs around him and kissing him passionately. Though he thought he wanted her, something about her boldness now bothered him and he gently pushed her off of him.

"Save that for later," he said and gave her peck.

If she was annoyed, he did not detect it, and instead she straightened herself up and headed for the living room. He checked his portfolio once more, memorizing the total value, and then headed out to join her.

Whatever the caterer was preparing smelled delicious and Colton realized how hungry he was. He circled around the coffee table eyeing the hors d'oeuvres. He snatched one up and popped it into his mouth. He poured himself a Scotch while he chewed. Cherie spied him at the bar and joined him, stopping first to pilfer a cheese-topped morsel for herself.

"Did you try the goat cheese?" she asked.

"No, the turnover," he replied. "Very good."

"Delicious, Brian," she called back to the chef in the kitchen. He bowed at the compliment.

"Where's he from?" Colton asked.

"Chez Georgeanne," she replied.

"Langford's favorite place," he said, startled.

"I'm well aware," she replied with a smile.

Colton kissed her on the forehead, genuinely impressed. Without even having to explain it to her, she understood how important this evening was.

The doorbell rang.

"Stay here. I'll get it," he said.

He ushered Langford and Patricia into the condo entryway and then into the living room where Cherie met them. Colton made all the proper introductions.

"Cherie, beautiful as always. What are you doing with this troll?" Langford asked.

Cherie looked shocked at the remark, but Colton just laughed it off. He knew Langford would trade these kinds of barbs, he also knew that the true measure of his judgment would be whether he stole inappropriate glances at Cherie. He intended to spend the evening watching how Langford looked at Cherie rather than eyeing up Patricia as he always did. Patricia looked more stunning than Colton remembered her, perhaps in contrast to his Cherie. The notion of that briefly agitated him. He believed Cherie to be beautiful from the moment he saw her. She was angular and dark, like his favorite type, while Patricia was pale and blond and more delicate, in spite of being a size bigger than Cherie.

"So, the holiday season's underway already," Langford said. "Seems like the Hamptons ended just yesterday, right? Oh sorry, I keep forgetting that you don't summer in the Hamptons, Colton. Well, not too much to miss."

"I met John Mayer on the beach," offered Patricia.

Colton saw Cherie light up at Patricia's celebrity sighting. He could see what Langford was doing; it was what Langford always did.

"You should come down to St Bart's sometime," he countered.

"The place is stunning!" Cherie gushed.

Langford polished off his drink and shook his glass for another. Colton poured a second drink and watched Langford shove a few more bites into his mouth.

"Well, winter's really the time for warm weather get-a-ways, don't you find? Took you down to the islands when you were a down-and-out student, didn't I, chump?" Langford lobbed.

"Don't remember," answered Colton.

"Cherie, poor guy here had to spend his winters in Michigan for a while. Worse than Philadelphia. Said he didn't even mind staying here while the rest of us took off, but I felt sorry for him, and dragged him along out of the kindness of my heart," said Langford.

Colton was trying to keep his cool, but Langford was worse than usual and showing off for Cherie. Thankfully, Cherie launched into a line of questions about Langford's business and Patricia's charity work that monopolized the conversation and gave Colton a break until dinner.

The conversation remained light during most of dinner, with Colton making sure that Langford's glass was always full. Cherie had done a perfect job choosing the menu. Each course was more delicious than the last, each course researched to make sure that it was either Langford or Patricia's favorite. After dinner, Colton excused himself from the table to retrieve the Balenciaga bag and he returned to hear Cherie chatting with Langford and Patricia about the Kammerly event.

"So, chump, we sure were impressed to see Cherie in action at Kammerly. I think even Daddy was impressed," he said.

Colton clutched. His father and Langford huddled together for most of the night, only breaking up to toss barbs his way. Now there would be more fallout that would make it even more painful.

"I'm surprised you could fit it into your schedule on such short notice," Colton said.

He flashed a look at Cherie and she drew back, puzzled. She should have known better than to participate in a conversation with Langford about last night. He fought the urge to become sullen.

"Oh, I almost forgot. I have something for you, Patricia. Cherie had been searching for these for some time, and I finally found them. I thought you might like a pair too," said Colton, watching for Langford's response.

Patricia opened the bag and spotted the jeans. Her face lit up immediately as she recognized the distinctive stitching and the nature of the gift. Without pulling them out of the bag for display, nor checking the size, she smiled at Colton and leaned over to give him a warm hug.

"Sale at the GAP?" Langford chuckled.

"Balenciaga jeans, Lang. Very tough to come by," Patricia snapped.

Langford drew back and shot a look at Patricia, and then turned his attention to Colton.

"Very nice, chump," he said.

"My pleasure," replied Colton.

Langford pinched up his face and finished another drink. Colton had shown up Langford, which brightened his mood.

"I'll have to return the favor, Cherie. Perhaps she would be interested in something from your designer friend, Patricia," he said.

"Oh yes, Molly Mills. Her new season comes out next week," she said.

"Sounds like a girl's day out. On me, of course," said Langford.

Colton was amused by Langford's attempt to recover, though he tried hard not to register it on his face. Instead, he relished the hug from Patricia and fantasized that it meant more than it did. That would have to do for now.

Chapter 5

Form FDA 3500A, Incidents #295, etc.:

...In the fall, the supply of flu vaccine was administered across the United States, approximately 100 million doses in all and 17 million more than in previous years. Yet, in spite of the increase in Americans receiving the vaccine, this flu season is predicted to be one of the worst on record, with upwards of almost 25,000 deaths attributed to the outbreak nationwide already. By the season's end, the United States may easily see deaths in the 100,000 range or higher, a level not seen since the late 1950s. While about a third of the deaths so far occurred in those who had not received a flu vaccine, another two thirds of those who died had received a flu vaccine within the timeframe recommended for effectiveness.

Quarantined samples from suspect lots were tested and found to contain little or no vaccine, but a large percentage of simple saline solution. Lots were traced to manufacturing facilities in China, India, the United Kingdom, and United States. Upon further investigation, it was determined that the vaccines were counterfeits designed to look like legitimate product from known facilities, but may actually have originated from a single facility deliberately engineering labels and packaging to mimic existing supply. Still searching for the source of the counterfeit vaccines, though the facility may have already been shut down when news of the epidemic reached the news media...

***

Sundays were Kat's only day to sleep in, and even Bernie respected that fact and managed to control himself until Kat was ready to get up and let him out. Unfortunately, Dan had called an emergency morning meeting for and so instead of lolling in bed, Kat was padding around her kitchen, grumbling about having to get up on a Sunday.

"Don't these guys realize that the Lord said it's a day off? Huh?" she asked Bernie, who was more interested in her morning breath than in the words that came out of her mouth.

She opened the back door and let him out into the yard to relieve himself while she put on a pot of coffee in the kitchen. They had only been home since Friday afternoon, but in that short amount of time, the two had already managed to thoroughly mess up most of the house. Something happened to Kat's finicky self on her trip to Philadelphia, something besides just sleeping with Jimmy, although that was a highpoint. Somehow that night had turned her into a different person, one who no longer found it necessary to keep her living quarters in spit polish shape, not that that had been completely possible with the addition of Bernie anyway. Just as she was relishing lounging in her mess yesterday, Maryanne had called.

"Dan's raging," she said.

"So, what else is new?" asked Kat.

"He wants all investigators in OCI tomorrow at 10a.m. sharp," Maryanne continued.

Dan was usually more of a hands-off kind of manager, content to read reports rather than call person-to-person meetings. The fact that he was calling an emergency meeting at the Office of Criminal Investigations, on a weekend no less, meant something grave. Kat let Bernie back in the house and left a note for the dog service to make sure to give him extra attention. Poor Bernie had to transition from an all-day attention party at Albe's frat house to life at home with just Mom, to being all alone. Kat shuttered to think of what that hound might get into if left to his own devices too long. She showered and dressed, wolfed down some breakfast, grabbed the bag with Dan's Tastykakes, and took off for OCI. As Kat pulled past security and spotted Maryanne in the parking lot, she beeped to signal for her to wait up. She parked the car and hurried over to catch up.

"Any clue?" Kat asked.

"Not much. I'm hearing rumblings about Senator Connelly blowing his stack and threatening to embarrass the department. Then I hear the opposite side where Dan is about to march up to Capitol Hill and bust a few knuckleheads himself," she said.

"Just on general principal or did something come in that I don't know about?" Kat asked.

"You know everything I know," Maryanne shrugged.

The conference room was already stacked with bleary-eyed and baffled investigators wondering why they were dragged to Rockville for a command performance on what was a peaceful Sunday. Thankfully, Dan or someone on his staff had thought ahead, providing a table with coffee and food. Kat was in dire need of more strong coffee to bolster her this morning. She listened to the conversation in the room as she poured her coffee and heard some rumblings that sounded too sensational to be true and, as usual, a lot of speculation, but no one seemed to have a definite clue. With her coffee in hand, Kat took up a place at the table and waited like the rest of the room.

"Let's get started," Dan announced as he walked in. Kat almost didn't recognize him dressed in relaxed and casual weekend wear. His demeanor was anything but. Without any niceties, he plunged right in.

"As of today, this department is in crisis mode. Over the past 72 hours, we've received hundreds of incident reports, more than the past five years *combined*. Concurrently, we're hearing from the CDC that they're tracking a number of instances of super bugs, heightened allergic reactions, and physicians reporting that they are seeing decreased efficacy in course of treatment. We've alerted Homeland Security and HHS Secretary Rogers, who will be on site in about an hour. The tech team is preparing the data and we should have the reports up soon. We're linking to all personnel worldwide via webcast and go over the scope of the problems. Questions?"

So much air was sucked out of the room from Dan's announcement that it took a moment for the agents to be able to breathe again. Kat knew now that sick feeling she'd been carrying in her gut was real, just the kind of thing you don't want to be right about. She pulled herself together, glanced around the room and stuck up her hand.

"What exactly are we dealing with here?" she asked.

"Not sure whether it's coincidental or deliberate," answered Dan.

"Casualties?" someone asked.

"Hundreds so far," he answered.

"Single drug?" someone else asked.

"No, multiple and across a broad spectrum," he replied.

There was an audible gasp in the room. Dan had made his point loud and clear.

"As soon as tech is ready to go, we're on," Dan finished and then strode out without taking any more questions.

A stunned silence hung over the room as investigators tried to process Dan's bombshell. It was unusual enough to receive that many MedWatch reports in such a short period, more unusual to hear of that many casualties at the same time. Everyone in the department knew that a certain percentage of prescription medications were counterfeit; the goal was to hold that number steady. But recently, the numbers had been progressively rising. Department speculation laid blame on a volatile mixture of more offshore manufacturing and fewer inspection resources, not to mention a more cozy relationship between the FDA and the drug manufacturers. This White House made no bones about the fact that it had little regard for government oversight and trusted the industry to police itself. Like everyone else in the department, Kat knew that profit was a more powerful motivator than morals. Still, with about four billion prescriptions filled each year, even these elevated numbers didn't seem like much, but the department's job was to act quickly enough, knowing how quickly hundreds could turn into thousands.

"Anybody hearing anything?" asked Chris, an investigator from Atlanta.

"Not enough information to go on. We're all seeing all kinds of things, right? Gotta narrow it down before we can figure it out," answered Nguyen, newest guy out of California.

The veterans of the group were more at ease than the new hires. They had seen a few of these resource-wide alerts over the years but even they were huddled together, chattering.

While the guys on the food safety side were almost used to these broader alerts and recalls, theirs had also been rising over the past few years. Drug side recalls usually involved labeling changes or warnings and not usually pulling the drug from shelves, with the exception of the recent Heparin recall. Clearly something grave was up and Kat was getting antsy like everyone else, knowing that her original suspicions were becoming a reality.

It was less than an hour before tech came into the room with equipment and boxes full of folders, one for each assembled investigator. Without waiting for them to be distributed, everyone crowded over to the boxes and retrieved a folder, then retired to a seat to pore over the information inside. Soon the room was eerily quiet, the only sound was of the tech crew setting up and testing the web cam and laptops for Dan and the other speakers.

Kat read through the opening report, trying to slow her pounding heart. The conclusion was tentative, but serious: "…reliable evidence that counterfeit drugs into the legitimate market are on the rise and the problem spans the spectrum of all drug classes. Further, the FDA is working closely with the CDC to investigate cases of resistant bacterial strains to determine whether loss of efficacy in antibiotics used to treat the infections is related to the presence of counterfeit drugs in the legitimate drug supply."

In other words, someone—and it had to be someone big judging by the scope of the reports—was compromising the entire legitimate drug supply with counterfeits. This was a bold new move. Up to this point, counterfeiters stayed in the Internet marketplace, bilking consumers directly. The web enterprises were lucrative and easily mobile. They had no storefront, no face-to-face, no on-sites, and when investigators got too close, they simply shut down, waited a few days, and opened up again under a new name. The big money drugs were the erectile dysfunction drugs like Viagra and Cialis, painkillers, and other drugs that might be of interest for "recreational" use. Now a new animal had been unleashed, a rabid dog that masqueraded as a family pet and Kat's head was spinning.

"Let's get started," Dan announced as he strode back into the room.

Investigators tore themselves away from their information packets and focused on the screen at the front of the room where Dan stood. Tech had linked in offices in China, England, India, and Puerto Rico with OCI. After each office introduced itself, division chief Roger Downes took the floor.

"The reports from England pre-date those from the U.S., but some of the cases are similar, specifically with classes of antibiotics and the diuretics."

"Findings?" Dan asked.

"Only that we've done exhaustive searches and testing of most of the manufacturing facilities and found nothing. The problem has been that not all the reported problems, or the range of the problems, occurred in a single lot."

Angel Munoz broke in. "Excuse me, Dan, we're seeing exactly the same thing at supply coming out of plants here in Puerto Rico." Kat had met Munoz at a conference last year, gaining enormous respect for him after he explained the need for increased pharmaceutical distribution to underserved nations.

"Same classes of drugs?" Dan asked.

"Yes, with one addition. There's some early evidence that the antiarrhythmics may be involved too."

Dan turned to address the investigators in the room.

"It appears that all of the drugs were sold in the U.S. market only, regardless of where they were manufactured. Mr. Chen, can you tell us your finings in China?"

Chen was a round faced, plump, middle-aged government official, responsible for China's pharmaceutical industry. Though he was dressed in western clothing, he reminded Kat of an elderly Chairman Mao.

"We have shut down one plant only that has been linked to the early cases of allergic reactions with the anti-inflammatory Vioxx, but that pre-dated these recent reports," said Chen.

"Now, in the Heparin case, you guys were dealing with deliberately substituted counterfeit product that was added so it would test out like the active ingredient," Dan said. "Any evidence that this is happened with other products?"

"No hard evidence yet, but that's the direction the investigation is headed," Mr. Chen answered.

"Is it likely that any of that raw produce made it way out of China to the States? Or are you focusing on finished product at your plants?" asked Dan.

"Both. We could be looking for export of raw materials to manufacturing facilities in countries other than the United States, where it may be easier to get adulterated product in the door. But we may be looking for a counterfeit finished product."

Another voice and face chimed in. "Dan, Balram Patel here. I had to weigh in. We are definitely looking for finished product and raw materials here in India. It is no secret that there is a great deal of activity in this market here, but we have not been able to link to the United States market except through Internet activity."

Patel was in the eye of the storm. No matter how hard his agency worked, the underground trade in India was a formidable opponent. It was almost as though Patel took the breaches personally. Kat wondered how a guy like that could even get up and do his job every day.

"When are we going to have more hard evidence," Dan asked. "This is for all of you."

"Should be a week," answered Roger first.

"Week to ten days," added Angel.

"Week, sure," said Chen.

"We will have some ideas," said Balram, "but a week is not nearly enough time.

Dan opened the floor to the investigators, who rapid-fired questions after question to each of the four officers. As the questions became repetitive, Kat's attention waned and she began rifling through the reports again, searching for anything that might make more sense. There just seemed to be too many drugs from too many manufacturers to suggest this was something at the manufacturing level. If it were at the raw materials level, then that was a lot of back door activity—too much in fact to make sense. Someone would have talked by now. It was not likely that multiple tests could have been faked or manipulated at that many facilities. It had to be in distribution. Question was what distributor would take the chance at moving counterfeit product? And how was it being done on such a scale? Judging by how widespread the problem was, the distributor must be big. That thought was the scariest of all. Kat went down the list of the biggest players in her area and realized the scope of the work ahead. Jimmy's name was on that list too, and suddenly her extracurricular activity struck her as an even bigger mistake that she first feared.

"Any more questions for international?" Dan asked as the questions finally died down.

"Thanks all. Keep us posted," he concluded and tech shut down the webcast.

Dan turned back to the investigators. Kat could see by the ashen color of his skin and the dark circles under his eyes that he was more concerned about this than he was even letting on. Dan was the kind of guy who took his work very seriously, which was how he ended up in the top spot at a relatively young age. It was also that he had a reputation as a straight shooter with his superiors and Congress but didn't come off as combative or arrogant. If anything, Dan's fault was that he cared too much and it was clearly taking its toll on his health. Suddenly, Kat felt guilty about the bag of Tastykakes and hoped that she could get out of the room without actually giving them to him.

"We have to mobilize in a different way on this one. We need more personnel in the field. I'm reassigning some of you into clusters to cover the facilities faster. Even though we're seeing a national involvement, we're going to start with the big three distributors, then their largest distributors, and so on. You'll find the cluster lists in the back of the folders."

There was lots of paper ruffling as the investigators took out the cluster lists and checked to see with whom they were working. Kat was assigned two investigators, one from Louisiana and one from West Virginia, neither of whom she had ever met before.

"Here's where we're going to start," Dan continued. "Teams will conduct an on-site at each manufacturer first and send samples to the lab for testing. If you've been on a site in the past week, there's no need to revisit, but include the sample testing in your research. Next, move to your large distributor first, then to his largest. What we know is that the scope of this is too big for a mom-and-pop, so it's got to be a bigger enterprise. The problem is we just don't know how big. On-site inspections, interviews, sample retrieval, logs, and financials. Don't forget the financials.

You can split up the work as you see fit but I need to make sure that all the bases are covered."

If the other investigators hadn't realized it yet, Kat knew that Dan was talking about an almost insurmountable amount of work. Even though ninety percent of all prescription drug wholesale distribution is conducted by three companies—NorthAmerica-Genberg in Pennsylvania, McCraken in California, and Bishop Health in Ohio—there could be hundreds of smaller distributors and any one of them could be responsible for the problem. Unfortunately, one of the big ones was right in Kat's front yard.

Of course, that would be the easy part, because the big guys are used to the FDA's visits, but it was what came after that would be the challenge. After the big boys were the regional wholesale drug distributors, of which there might be 15 to 20. Probably half of those were in Kat's region. Then would come the biggest headache of all: inspecting the estimated 6,000 to 7,000 smaller drug wholesalers. Kat had no idea how many of those were hers. The only saving grace was that the smallest of the distributors operated primarily in niche markets, servicing dispensing physicians and small pharmacies, dispensers in rural areas, and buyers of specialty drugs that require special handling. All of that was much easier to trace.

"Excuse me, Ma'am. Are you Ms. Vasquez?" asked a white-haired, rotund elder gentleman.

"Call me Kat. Nice to meet you…" she said as she stood to shake hands.

"Lonny Star, from West Virginia. Pleasure to meet you."

Lonny took a firm grip on her hand and shook it for what seemed like too long of a time.

"How long you been with the department, Lonny?" she asked.

"Oh, goin' on 'bout ten years now. Got in after I sold my pharmacy," he said.

"Kat?" asked a young man who had made his way from the far side of the room.

"Tyrell Blackberry. The only fly in the buttermilk here," he said.

The joke made everyone else uncomfortable and Tyrell was the only one that laughed. Kat held out her hand and shook his, then introduced him to Lonny Star.

"So, I guess it's the three of us now," said Kat.

"I see here that NorthAmerican-Genberg is in your area, along with some of the largest distributors. Think we need to ask for more help?" Lonny wiped his brow as though just thinking about the amount of work ahead made him sweat.

"I don't know about you, but I can hit a facility and get a beat in a short time. Just gotta talk to the right folks, you know?" said Tyrell.

"NorthAmerican-Genburg has a few locations in this area, but we'll start with the largest. Then move on to the next tier of distributors," said Kat.

"You live in that area?" asked Lonny.

"No. I'll give you the name of place I usually stay. In fact, maybe the first thing is to book the rooms," said Kat.

She checked her watch and saw that it was still early enough in the day to head to Philadelphia. After getting the okay from both Lonny and Tyrell, she booked three rooms at the Holiday Inn Express in West Philadelphia. Then she called Albe, who agreed to take Bernie again for a few days.

"I gotta stop home and get packed and grab the dog," she announced. "Anybody got a rental car?"

Both Lonny and Tyrell had rentals, so Kat pulled quick directions for them from HQ to the hotel and three split up, agreeing to meet for dinner at the hotel. Kat packed up her things and was about to head out the door when Dan called her over.

"Since you're one of the three regions with the big guys, I'm putting three more investigators out there with you," Dan said. "Don't worry—they have a specific list of second tier wholesalers that aren't on your lists. I don't need you all tripping over one another in the field. Here are the briefs on what they'll be working on. These are seasoned people, so you don't have to supervise day-to-day. Just act as point person for the region."

"Thanks, Dan," she said and tried to scurry out the door.

"And, ah, you got my Tastykakes?" he asked before she got two more steps.

She couldn't help but flash a look at his bulging belly and quickly decide whether she wanted to be party to his health problems or not.

"I, ah—" she stumbled.

"Hey, anyone forget a bag here?" called someone from the back of the room.

"Over here," Kat called back, looking at Dan apologetically for her alleged forgetfulness. The man from the back brought her the bag with the Tastykakes, which she handed over to Dan.

"Don't worry, I'm sharing with the family," he said, smiling. "Promise."

With that, he took off out the door with his briefs and his bag of Tastykakes. Kat waited a moment before she followed. By the time she left the conference room, most of the investigators were on their way to their respective territories in search of whoever it was that was poisoning America. Kat was so busy mobilizing and thinking of sheer logistics that the gravity of the situation she would be in for the next few days or weeks or months until this case was solved didn't hit her until she was heading north to Philadelphia on I-95 with Bernie soundly snoring in the back.

She was conflicted about being assigned additional investigators, preferring instead to move at her own pace with her own ideas. She had walked away from a supervisory job on purpose, preferring solitude and autonomy to managing personalities. She could see that Lonny and Tyrell may not make the best team, good ole white boy from West Virginny and a southern black guy from New Orleans. Maybe too much diversity and a little too much assumed history. Kat groaned out loud. She couldn't wait to see what the other investigators were like. Still, there was just too much for one person to handle under normal circumstances, let alone an expanding crisis. Unfortunately, the FDA did not have enough regulators to monitor all the manufacturers and distributors on a regular basis, nor did it have laws with enough bite to control the current globalization of the drug marketplace. A 2006 FDA report concluded that 80 percent of the active pharmaceutical ingredients used in prescription drugs in the United States were imported from abroad. Only 32 field inspections were made in India and 15 in China, the two largest sources of ingredients.

Still, even if she found the creeps, Kat had no power to prosecute. All she could do was impose fines and arrange for shameful headlines. If she wanted to have the perpetrators shut down, she had to bring in the FBI and local law enforcement to uncover tax evasion or interstate trafficking or other applicable broken laws. Problem was, she couldn't tip off those agencies until she finished her own investigations, and by that time, the FBI and local guys often had a huge attitude. Kat groaned aloud again and this time Bernie imitated her.

The only law the department could use to control counterfeit drugs was the Prescription Drug Marketing Act of 1987 (PDMA), but since 1988 the FDA had been unable to enforce the major provisions of the law, primarily because of pressure from the wholesale drug distributors. Every wholesaler was supposed to be able to provide a pedigree for every drug distributed, submitting a set of paperwork that vouched for every sale of the drug before the sale made by the wholesaler. The problem was that the PDMA exempted those "authorized distributors of record" or the distributors with whom a manufacturer had established an "ongoing relationship" to distribute product. It was a loophole large enough to drive a tractor-trailer full of drug through. Wholesale distributors cried foul and refused to comply with the provisions and the teeth were cut right out of the law.

While the FDA and wholesalers continued to argue over who had to produce the pedigree papers, Kat and all the other inspectors watched more and more counterfeits stream into the marketplace and more and more people get sick and die.

Her jaw tensed up from frustration over the powerlessness of politics. She turned her attention to where she did have control through the investigation. Why would NorthAmerican-Genburg, or any manufacturer, commit such a crime? It just didn't seem likely that any of the big players would chance moving counterfeits or that any of the mucky mucks in the company would risk their position. As illogical as it seemed, she still thought it was a big mistake to dismiss any possibilities, since oftentimes the least likely answer was the true scenario. She had to think like someone who deliberately decided to infuse counterfeits into their supply line. She had to think like the guys she was chasing. First question was why: why do it?

It was no secret that even the big wholesalers sometimes moved expired goods through the marketplace, accidentally maybe, or in an effort to unload them and hope that the dates weren't checked often enough for them to get caught. It was easy enough to claim a mistake and take the supply back but the unspoken hope was that no one checked expiration dates. Counterfeits were a completely different animal—much more deliberate, much less easy to defend to yourself. Something had happened in the last few years that made them explode into the legitimate marketplace. Either wholesalers were unaware that they were buying counterfeits or they knew full well and were willing to take the chance at not getting caught for a little extra bump in the profits. Both possibilities raised goose bumps on Kat's arms.

***

Colton ran down the list in his head and checked off every last item. He'd been systematically testing Cherie since he'd met her, keeping tabs on how she measured up to each of his criteria. As she passed each new test, Colton neared the day that he would ask her to marry him. He grappled with his doubts, but once he saw her in action at the Kammerly auction, and then how she deftly handled Langford and Patricia, he was convinced that it was time to propose. It didn't hurt that Joe Daddy loved her either, not that Colton wanted to care.

He had asked her to move in with him only months after they first met but then turned cautious and worried whether he had made a mistake. That's when he created his list. First, he exposed her to some of his business dealings; nothing too revealing, just enough that a smart girl could guess the true nature of his business and test if she was willing to ignore it for the rewards that would follow. Cherie never registered even a hint of distaste. In St. Bart's especially, she easily fit in with the schedule of the day and seemed content. She never snooped into his things in the condo, even when he deliberately left them out as a test. She never asked where he was going or when he would be returning, instead only expressing how much she missed him and how much she hoped he would have time for her. Maybe someday someone as accomplished as Cherie would grow tired of the arrangement, but the longer he knew her, the more easily he brushed away those fears. He wasn't sure what it was about her—maybe her days at the conservatory, maybe that she had never pursued her concert career—but Cherie just seemed to accept whatever being with him entailed. He was good to her, he showered her with gifts and appreciation, and he found ways to control his other side.

The first time he saw Cherie at work, he worried that she was not right for him at all. She was a woman in charge, in control, always on top of her underlings, not at all the kind of woman Colton wanted next to him in her personal life. But the more he got to know her, the more he discovered that she, like him, had the unique ability to split herself into two people, knowing precisely which one needed to be present and when.

For the first time in his life, he wanted to please a woman and wanted a full-time companion. He surprised her with the Baldwin grand piano she had been saving for, the one she had talked about since they met. She crumbled into a heap of slobbering tears when she saw it, and he too was overcome with emotion. He had the piano placed in the corner of the living room of the condo, the north corner that faced the Kammerly Center where the floor-to-ceiling windows allowed the light in the atrium dome to glow in the background. It made Cherie happy and it was something he could point out to Langford the next time he chided him for not buying on Rittenhouse Square.

Colton loved to watch Cherie play. She was accomplished and strong. He was captivated by the way she moved as she expertly touched the keys. He fantasized about her sitting naked at the piano and playing, with the drapes open and the only light in the room emanating from the Kammerly Center atrium. He imagined his Cherie naked before the city, with only him being able to see her. He even told her about his fantasy once, halfway confessing, halfway testing. At first she just blushed, smiled and kissed him. Then, one day, she surprised him by acting it out. It was better than he had imagined. The real feel and smell of Cherie made his fantasy even better. He knew then that he could trust her and love her completely.

He had started to send signals to Cherie lately that maybe he might be interested in marriage by mentioning the future, talking about family and kids, and even once taking her through Caldwell's to look at jewelry. She invited him to meet her family and he dutifully traveled to Lancaster County with her, even wearing his best disposition the entire day. He laughed at her father's stupid jokes and admired her mother's assortment of Pennsylvania Dutch tchotchkes, ate her mother's country food and generally behaved himself. The entire day became less agonizing when he discovered that her father was the president of Farmstead Bank. He contemplated how useful that might become in the future.

He had already scaled the mountain of introducing Cherie to his bastard father and his judgmental mother. He had been careful and calculating about the meeting. Two things he knew from experience with his parents: it was important to keep his father in a place where he felt none too comfortable and without any hard liquor, and, two, to exploit his mother's tendency to be overly compensating by creating some kind of incident that made her want to mother him.

He had booked dinner at Bon, one of the notable BYOBs in the Philadelphia suburbs run by a chef who had cut his teeth at the five-star Le Bec Fin. Colton bought two bottles of impressive but not ostentatious wine, knowing full well that his father was lost without his beloved whiskey. Then he pre-arranged for Reggie to interrupt their dinner with some urgent business crisis, which he solved before their very eyes.

Cherie so skillfully charmed his parents that he momentarily thought he didn't need his plan. He quickly dismissed that thought when his father needled him with a jibe about not qualifying for his college football team, followed by the inevitable bragging about his younger brother who consistently made all-American and now played for the Seattle Seahawks. Although Colton thought the evening went as well as it could have for an evening with his parents, it still left him on edge. Somehow, Cherie instinctively knew he was wounded and when they returned to the condo, spent the rest of the evening making up for the humiliations he suffered.

When Colton ran down his entire list, he realized that Cherie was much more of a woman he wanted than he had first imagined. He would ask her to marry him and to seal the deal he bought a four-carat diamond and platinum ring, a full carat bigger than the one Langford gave to Patricia. He would present it to her tonight, during dinner. He was picking up his new suit when he began worrying that

Jackie Jr. had once again messed up another job he had been assigned.

"Jackie, did you confirm the reservations?" he asked.

Colton was too nervous to drive and had insisted that Jackie come out from his suburban dump to drive him around and keep him company. Cherie was working today, a children's Meet the Musician Day at the Kammerly, so he had time to run some last minute errands and get the condo ready for his evening of surprises.

"I made them, but I didn't confirm them," he replied.

"Get on the phone and confirm them while I'm in getting fitted," he barked. It was exasperating to have to constantly follow up after Jackie and Colton often thought about how much easier it would be to just get rid of him.

"You're nervous, huh?" asked Jackie.

"Excited maybe." Colton didn't want Jackie to know that he could even be nervous.

"You're doing the right thing," Jackie offered.

"Glad I got your approval," Colton snapped.

"I didn't mean it that way. I just meant that Cherie's a great girl, someone you don't want to let go of. Does she know, you know, about, ah… everything?" he asked.

"You think I'm stupid? Why would you even ask me that?" he shot.

"I don't know, I just thought because she's all society and everything, that—" Jackie stammered.

"That she wouldn't be wasting her time with someone like me?" Colton barked.

Colton could see Jackie twitching, like always.

"No, no. That maybe she wouldn't understand, you know

"Since when did you become some kind of society guy, huh," he shouted. "When you married that South Philly mob daughter? That piece of shitloudmouth? Huh? She make you into a society guy? Not that you deserve an explanation, but Cherie understands everything exactly. You think I'm some kind of stupid?"

Colton slammed his hand on the dashboard. Jackie was always like that, stating the obvious, assuming that he was the smartest one in the room. Colton clenched his jaw. Jackie had a way of making him as small as he felt in college as the butt of the jokes and the recipient of Jackie and Langford's superior attitudes. He exited the car and slammed the door without another word. Now he wasn't going to enjoy his fitting because of Jackie and he huffed in the door, allowing it to slam behind him.

Luigi's wife greeted him cheerfully. "Ciao, Mr. Barnes! I bring you cappuccino! Your favorite!"

She led him into the sitting area outside the dressing room and he sat down on the overstuffed chair. She reappeared moments later with a steaming cup and biscotti, which she sat on the table beside him.

Then Luigi burst into the room. "Mr. Barnes! You will be very happy I hope," he said in his heavy Italian accent.

Colton needed some time to calm himself down after Jackie so he waved him off.

"Sure, sure. You enjoy. I take you in when you want, okay?" Luigi backed out of the dressing room.

Colton dipped the biscotti into his cappuccino and took a bit, lingering over the taste, willing himself to calmness. It took many more sips. Meanwhile, Luigi and his wife scurried around the workroom waiting for the right moment to debut their work. Colton loved picking up his custom suits, loved the way Luigi perfectly tailored them to fit him, and especially loved the way they made him feel. He did not want his experience ruined by thoughts of Jackie. Finally, Colton stood up. Luigi and his wife swooped over and ushered him into the dressing room along with his suit. He admired how good it looked just hanging on the hanger. He changed into it and stood in front of the mirror turning this way and that, twisting and admiring himself from every direction. He stepped out from the dressing room and stood in front of the three-way mirror where Luigi waited. He hadn't noticed it before, but in the three-way mirror Colton saw the slight bulge of the additional pounds he had accumulated lately and frowned.

"You see something you no like? I fix. I fix," Luigi said, picking and pulling at the suit jacket.

"No, no Luigi. It's beautiful," he said.

"Oh, Mr. Barnes, you look like the royalty!" Mrs. Ciccio gushed.

Colton stared at the bulge, sucked in his gut, turned from side to side, examined the difference, and then unbuttoned the jacket.

Luigi brought over a custom-made peach shirt and another in pale green, both of which complimented the dark brown, pinstriped suit perfectly.

"This blue is beautiful with. I make two more in colors I think you like too," said Luigi.

"The blue's good for now," he said.

Colton liked the blue shirt best; it played perfectly off his blue eyes and helped him look sincere. Luigi and his wife continued to flutter around Colton, cooing and admiring how the suit looked.

"You like?" Luigi finally asked.

"Very nice work," Colton replied.

The two let out an audible sigh and Mrs. Ciccio rushed off declaring that he should have a special Ciccio garment bag to take his suit home.

Colton changed back into his clothes and left the suit and shirt in the room for Luigi to retrieve. Moments later, at the front of the store, his suit and shirts were all properly packed into a garment bag and the Ciccio's waited for payment. Colton pulled out his wallet and paid Luigi in cash, adding a few hundred dollar bills for a tip. Both Luigi and his wife walked him out to the car and the man carefully hung the garment bag from the hook inside the back seat of the truck. They waited until Colton got into the truck and waved to him as Jackie pulled away from the curb.

"The reservation?" Colton asked.

"Eight o'clock, confirmed," he replied.

"Why did I have to ask? Why didn't you just know to tell me when I got into the car?" Colton shot.

"Sorry, I—" Jackie stammered.

"You know, I must hear that a dozen times a day from you. If you didn't fuck up in the first place, you would have to say sorry all the time!" Colton shouted.

"Sor—"

"Shut the fuck up and get me over to the office."

Colton saw Jackie snap his head around to look at him.

"The office?" he asked.

Colton leaned over closer to Jackie and asked, "You got a problem with that? I got a meeting in fifteen minutes."

"Oh. You think you're gonna be long?" Jackie said with a hint of a whine in his voice.

"Why?" Colton asked.

"Wife wants me to be there for Mikey's first soccer game today," Jackie responded, nearly inaudibly.

Colton could never understand why Jackie put up with being ordered around by his loudmouth wife. She didn't seem to understand that Jackie worked for him and not her, but then Jackie never put her in her place either, except one time when she opened her big mouth at Colton and Jackie had clocked her one across the face. Colton still thought about that whenever he saw her.

"Just drop me at the condo. I'll take my own car," Colton said with as much disgust in his voice as he could muster.

"Sorry, Col—"

"Save it, Jackie. Tonight's too important for me to waste time getting aggravated by you again today."

Jackie made his way through the Center City traffic and finally over to Broad Street, where he dropped Colton off in front of Symphony House. Colton handed his garment bag to the doorman and asked him to put it in his condo, tipping him fifty bucks for his trouble. Then he took the elevator down to the parking garage and retrieved his Escalade to head out to Malvern for his meeting.

There were only a few cars in the parking lot when Colton arrived at the office; he only needed a skeleton crew on Saturdays. He punched in the security code and opened the door and made his way to his office in the back where he turned on the lights and made himself comfortable in his chair. This was Jackie Sr.'s old office. Colton got rid of Jackie's tacky South Philly décor and completely redecorated with mahogany desk and bookcases, leather couch and chairs, and fine wool carpeting. He felt at home and powerful in the extravagant room and it helped him get over his nagging fear that though he was brilliant at his own enterprise, he wasn't smart enough to run USA Distributors.

He poured himself a short Scotch at the bar, downed it relishing the burn, and waited for the call about his meeting. It was only moments before his cell rang and he made his way to the front door of the building.

"You find us okay?" he asked.

"No problem," answered Jimmy Kirk.

Colton had been thinking about expanding and wasn't quite sure how to proceed. Seeing Jimmy at the Kammerly Center auction the other night was like a revelation. He and Jimmy and his partners traveled in some of the same circles, sharing information that could be mutually beneficial and often meeting up at some event or another, wooing the very same clients. They were cordial competitors, each finding their niche in a particular facet of the market and overwhelmed enough with their own business issues to prevent them from becoming too adventurous into each another's. Distributors often borrowed product from one another, particularly when the manufacturers caused supply shortages. In fact, grousing about pharmaceutical manufacturers was pretty much a common ground among distributors and consumers alike.

Colton walked Jimmy to his office and offered him a drink, which Jimmy refused. Colton sat down behind his expansive desk in his executive chair that was deliberately set higher than the other chairs in the room. He read once that to gain an edge in business, you needed to insure that you were larger than life to others. Jimmy was a good few inches taller than Colton, but sitting in Colton's office would make him feel physically smaller.

"Good to see you the other night. You bid on anything?" Colton began.

"A few things," Jimmy said, quickly adding, "It was a great event though, great night."

"The auctioneer is Cherie, my fiancée. She runs that every year," Colton said proudly.

"Great job. Beautiful woman," Jimmy replied.

"So, who did I see you with there? The brunette?" he probed.

"Nah, I was alone," Jimmy replied.

Colton eyed him closely, watching him fidget. He figured that Jimmy was lying and wondered why.

Colton changed the subject, leaning back in his chair. "So, I'll just plunge right in. You got two partners in the business with you?"

"Why?" Jimmy shifted so that he sat solidly in the chair.

Colton casually waved his hand, "Just trying to get the lay of the land."

"I've got partners, yes,"

"How invested are you? I mean, personally?" asked Colton.

Jimmy chuckled and shifted in his seat again.

"Look, Colton, I'm all for sharing and all that, but you got to tell me what you're driving at here, 'cuz I just may get offended that you think I would be a disloyal kind of guy."

Colton was testing to see how far he could go and in what direction. Now he knew Jimmy was the upstanding type and would probably choose loyalty and righteousness over plain old greed and power. Not that that would dissuade him from pursuing his course; he just have to play Jimmy differently to win.

"I didn't mean anything disrespectful, Jimmy. Just some innocent questions," he replied.

"And?"

"I was looking at the numbers and see that nursing homes and home care is expanding probably faster than any other part of the market," Colton continued.

"And?" Jimmy gripped the arm of the chair with his right hand.

"I'm not telling you anything you don't already know. You guys have a huge presence in that marketplace, lots of good friends, kind of where you're making your mark, huh?" Colton pressed.

Jimmy sighed and sat forward, looking Colton right in the eyes.

"C'mon Colton—what's the point?"

Colton stayed back in his chair, relaxed and comfortable. "Point is, maybe we could talk a deal here."

Jimmy chuckled, sitting back in his chair silently for a minute. "Depends on what kind of a deal," he finally said.

"Not sure. Merger, buyout...what do you think your guys would go for?" Colton asked.

"We aren't looking to go for anything at all," Jimmy replied.

"Everybody's got to have an exit strategy," Colton said. "You didn't get into this to stay in it the rest of your life. You got in it to imagine yourself retired by your mid-fifties, lounging on a beach somewhere, screwing a gorgeous twenty-something."

He could see Jimmy stewing on what he just said, trying to cut through his distrust and feel the possibility of the good life he described. This would be a tough sell, but it would certainly be easier to buy the exclusive relationships he needed rather than trying to build them. It was tough enough handling the production issue with the Chinese; now he was impatient to just get what he wanted the fast way.

"What are you getting at?" Jimmy blurted out.

"I'm pretty sure you figured it out," Colton replied.

"You understand we may not be as big as you, but we're a lucrative enterprise."

"If you're wondering whether I know how much it's going to cost me, the answer's yes," Colton said, leaning forward. "And I am prepared to pay it, provided the price is fair."

Jimmy stared at him now, unwavering. Colton kept his gaze even and his expression neutral, allowing Jimmy to take all the time he needed to feel assured that he was not blowing smoke. Jimmy finally spoke. "Listen Colton, I'm—"

Colton held up the palm of his hand. "No need for answers today. I just wanted to toss something out there and see where it goes from there. I've got plenty of time here and so do you."

He got up from his chair and walked to the door, holding it open. Jimmy stood up and exited, with Colton following. At the exit, they parted company and got in their respective cars. Whatever Jimmy was feeling about his meeting with Colton, he was keeping it inside. He didn't utter another word, not even a goodbye, cordial or otherwise. Colton knew that just tossing out a proposal was enough to get under someone's skin and enough to eventually bring them back to him. He would just have to wait.

He had first contemplated the buyout of Global Med Distributors the year before, but that was when the Heparin crisis broke. He wanted to stay put until he saw how tough the FDA could get, worried about what kind of additional scrutiny everyone was under. He decided it was better to just lay low and not do anything that might grab a headline. But the FDA, though swift in isolating the source of the adulteration once it finally came to their attention, remained blissfully unaware of the complete scope of the counterfeits in the marketplace. The only guys who got caught were too greedy, too fast. They only moved counterfeit product, which made them too easy to detect. He had long ago figured out that the key to success was mixing counterfeits with legitimate drugs, which meant fewer reactions, and less cause for worry. And he could operate legitimately. He could also control the profit margin by the amount he chose to mix into every shipment. If he felt there was too much scrutiny, he pulled back entirely, allowing nothing but legitimate drugs to hit the market. When he knew the FDA was otherwise occupied, he cut his legitimate stock with more counterfeit and then only with drugs that were least likely to draw any kind of adverse reaction, like the antihypertensives, cholesterol-lowering drugs, diuretics, allergy meds, painkillers, and even some of the antibiotics. By mixing counterfeits in with legitimates, he wouldn't take away anyone's drug entirely, just subject them to a subtherapeutic dose. The beauty was that subtherapeutic dosing was hard to determine and patients had to be affected for a long time in order for any suspicion to fall on their medications, if ever, and Colton knew that well. He was careful with the antibiotics since that could allow for resistant strains of bacteria and though that meant selling more expensive and profitable antibiotics, it also meant scrutiny as labs tried to isolate the resistant strain. The antibiotics needed careful control and Colton didn't always feel like paying that much attention, no matter how much following the news stories about how doctors struggled to find the right antibiotic to cure the current outbreak of whatever amused him. But he did have some lines he refused to cross. He never touched birth control pills or erectile dysfunction drugs. That was just cruel.

When the Heparin story broke, the government estimated that counterfeits constituted about 8 to 10 percent of the worldwide market. Colton laughed out loud when he heard that on CNN, knowing that his portion alone was approaching 25 percent, with plans to ramp up every year. Moving into nursing homes meant even bigger profits and very little scrutiny. It was lucrative business supplying substandard drugs to those that America had cast off already. Families only showed up intermittently and worried more about how to continue paying Mom's bill than whether her medication was legitimate. Doctors were hardly ever around to treat patients and there were too few nurses on staff. The nurses on staff were generally overworked and the nurse's aides were too dumb to spot a drug issue. It was his latest revelation that the way that America chose to treat its elderly could translate into huge profits. And it was just the beginning, because the first wave of the baby boomers was on its way to nursing homes soon. Colton was excited at the prospect of taking over this market.

He knew Jimmy would take his offer back to his partners. The three would refuse at first, and then they would eventually come around to talk more. It was just a matter of time before Colton got his way.

Chapter 6

Form FDA 3500A, Incident #121,365, etc.:

... In the fall of 2007, numerous hospital emergency rooms across Maryland, Virginia, Delaware, North Carolina, Washington D.C., Pennsylvania, and New Jersey reported a sharp increase in the occurrence of stroke victims. About 30 percent of victims were out of the previously accepted age range established by prior data clusters. The family member of one Maryland physician suffered a stroke at the age of 32. The physician, familiar with FDA reports of an increase in counterfeit drugs infiltrating the U.S. supply, had his family member's hypertension medication tested. Initial test results revealed that the active ingredient in the calcium channel blocker, amlodipine, was merely a fraction of what the tablet should have contained and that the tablet primarily consisted of inert components.

The physician quickly contacted hospital emergency rooms in surrounding states to find out whether any other testing of drug from affected patients had been conducted. In 100 percent of cases where medications were tested, they presented the same results. The manufacturer was temporarily shut down and all lots and logs reviewed; no adulterated medications were found. Conclusion was that the counterfeit medications had infiltrated the supply, although the source has yet to be identified.

***

Kat's phone rang and she fumbled around to answer it without flipping the truck on I-95. She was deep in thought from the morning's meeting at HQ, feeling the pressure of the work ahead.

"Hey, I tried your home number, but no answer," came Jimmy's cheerful voice.

Kat was both excited and dismayed to hear from him. What they shared just a few days ago, Kat's coming out of mourning as it were, was spectacular, but Kat knew all too well the danger of having that kind of relationship with a guy who owned a wholesale drug distributorship, especially now. Neither one of them could risk the consequences of that becoming public knowledge.

"I'm out in the field," she said.

"On a Sunday?"

Kat winced and fumbled around for an excuse that would make sense.

"Ah, you know how it is, always being under staffed. Just got to make my numbers by the end of the month," she lied.

"I'm going to be in Maryland on business on Tuesday and it would be great to see you again…"

Kat didn't know what to say now. Of course it would be great to see him and she desperately wished she could, but she knew she had to put an end to it.

"Oh, ahhhh, I've got to go out of town for a few days, so I won't be there when you're there." Kat winced as she delivered the lie.

"I'm disappointed," he quickly replied.

"Yeah, me too," she mumbled.

Kat tapped her nails on the steering wheel to fill the awkward silence. Finally, Jimmy spoke.

"Kat, I meant what I said the other night. You are the first woman since my divorce I could envision myself with for the rest of my life."

Kat almost drove off the road when he said that. She had to tell herself not to speak for fear that she would say exactly the wrong thing. She could not describe her excitement at having found someone after Jorge, something she had convinced herself would never happen, yet that was tempered by the sadness that she would have to let the possibility of this relationship go forever.

"Kat, you there?" he asked.

"I'm here. I just don't know what to say," she replied.

"You don't have to say anything now. Listen, I'll call you tomorrow, okay?" said Jimmy.

"Sure. Tomorrow."

Then, he was gone, and Kat told herself it would be the last time she would ever speak to him in a non-professional context. Much as it pierced her heart to do so, from now on she had to check her caller ID and avoid Jimmy. She could moan and wail at the unfairness of the circumstance, and she probably would someday, but for now, she just wanted to cut off the hurt before it got any greater.

She pulled up in front of Albe's frat house about an hour later and her sleepy son, dressed in pajama bottoms and a T-shirt, sauntered out to retrieve Bernie. The two of them made the perfect picture. She fleetingly considered letting Bernie live with Albe full time.

"Back so soon, huh?" Albe asked.

"Don't know how long I have to be here, may be as long as a month. Maybe longer," she replied.

Albe seemed to guess the gravity of the situation either from her face or the length of time she thought she would be in town. He knew all too well that even her toughest case rarely took her more than a few days to complete.

"What's going on?" he asked.

"You know I can't answer," she said.

"I know. But when you can, let me know, huh? You look like you need someone to talk to," he said.

His face resembled Jorge's more and more, with his angular features and heavy beard. Only his light brown eyes looked like hers.

"I'm going to be tied up a lot but I'll come visit as much as I can," she said, turning her face away. She didn't want him to see the tears welling up in her eyes.

"Bernie'll be fine," he said. "Will you?"

Kat just nodded, said goodbye to Bernie, and got back in the truck. Then she paused and lowered the window.

"Hey," she called to Albe, who had only made it halfway to the front door, "Did I tell you how much I loved Martha?"

He smiled. "Did I?"

With that, she hurriedly pulled away, heading around the corner and up the few blocks to the hotel's underground garage. Once parked, she heaved a heavy sigh and sat for a while, thinking of how much her life had changed in the past few years and how little it resembled the life she thought it would be. The plan was that she and Jorge would be traveling the world by now, enjoying the second season of their lives together. They would start in Mexico, and then go on to South America. Next would be Spain, tracing the roots of his heritage, then through Western Europe. The next year would be Greece and Turkey and maybe even parts of the Middle East, if they felt safe. After that they had to decide whether it would be Africa or the Asian countries and the list would continue until they had made their way through the entire world and had seen and learned what they could about all of its peoples and cultures and lessons and lives. They would have endless conversations and endless memories and would feel like their lives were complete. Instead, Kat was alone and thinking about dating and not even thinking about a trip around the world. The worst part was there only seemed to be adolescent words to describe it all, words like dating and boyfriend, words without the dignity of her age. She didn't regret sleeping with Jimmy—in fact it opened up her world again—but she wasn't quite sure she was ready for that world. Yet, retreating seemed like trying to erase a thought you already had.

Finally, Kat exited the truck with her bags and the gravity of the situation hit her in a flash. The task ahead was formidable and the outcome would be tragic on a number of levels, there was no escaping that. As much as she wanted to solve this case, she couldn't deny the nagging feeling that she just wanted to run back in time to when things seemed much less complicated. She checked her watch after she grabbed her key from the front desk and decided she had just enough time drop her stuff off in the room before meeting with her new team in the lobby bar.

"I need a drink before I can get into all of this. How 'bout you all? You need a drink?" asked Tyrell.

He motioned for the waitress. To save time, the three decided to stay and eat at the hotel restaurant, which was a somewhat shabby and dark diner. The food was passable but at least the diner bragged of a well-stocked bar. Kat figured it was either to help travelers find their courage or numb themselves. The waitress greeted them sweetly and waited for their order.

"I'll have a strawberry daiquiri," began Tyrell.

"Bourbon, neat," added Lonny.

"You got a good Pino Noir?" Kat asked. The waitress nodded and Kat ordered a glass, knowing that it would be mediocre at best. She really wanted something stronger, but knew she needed to go slow. The waitress left and the three of them settled into their seats.

"So, what's the plan for tomorrow?" asked Tyrell.

He was a skinny, twitchy kind of guy. Pushy. He already irritated Kat, although she knew his energy would be extremely useful. She also knew he was going to be tough to control and tough to get to keep his mouth shut. On the other hand, Lonny seemed too laid back, too removed. Kat wondered whether she could get anything helpful out of him. The waitress reappeared almost immediately with the drinks before scurrying off. Kat took a sip of her wine. It was passable. Then, got down to business.

"I know it's already been a long day, but we need to go over the NorthAmerican-Genberg information so we're prepared for a Blitzkrieg tomorrow," said Kat.

"A what, what?" asked Tyrell.

"Blitzkrieg. We have to move fast. Hit hard and move on. Put them off-guard and sweep through before they can mobilize and ramp up the PR machine. The largest facility is not far from the corporate offices, but there are three other distribution sites across the state. We'll split into focus areas, solid dosage, sterile products and paperwork, including financials. Pick," said Kat at both of them at the same time.

Lonny and Tyrell sipped their drinks and pondered for a moment. Or, rather, Lonny pondered while Tyrell looked nervous and waited for Lonny to pick first.

"I, myself, am the kind of guy who shoots best with his old, familiar shotgun," Lonny finally announced.

Kat shook her head, squinting at him. She had no idea what he was talking about.

"I'm most comfortable with solid dosage," he clarified, "if that's okay with you Tyrell."

"No, no problem. So, Kat, you want me on sterile products or paperwork?" asked Tyrell.

Kat knew immediately that Tyrell would have no patience with paperwork, but was glad to see that he seemed to know himself well enough to know that too.

"Sterile products," she nodded.

"You got it. You got it. Sterile it is for me," he said.

Tyrell nervously sipped at his drink and Kat wondered whether he had ever conducted an inspection this huge and this detailed. But, she had to have confidence in Dan, who still kept his hand in every hire and paid close attention to all of his inspectors to ward off any coziness, like the guys over at the FAA. "Either you believe all guys are bad guys," Dan would say in his annual speech, "Or you believe there are no bad guys. Either way, you're wrong."

Kat opened her briefcase and handed a map of the NorthAmerican-Genberg facility to each of them and a checklist for their inspection tomorrow, broken down by area. The waitress interrupted them to take their dinner order. The wine had gone directly to Kat's head and then it hit her that she hadn't eaten since the morning.

After ordering, they went back to work.

"So, what kind of stripes this tiger got?" Lonny asked.

Again, Kat shook her head at him, baffled by his unique language. She looked at Tyrell who just shrugged and looked back at Lonny.

"What do you think is the real story here?" Lonny asked.

"What do you mean?" asked Kat.

"Somebody in there angling to make some money on the side, or the whole place full of snakes?" he said.

"I think it's dangerous to go in the door with conclusions," said Kat, knowing full well that it was impossible.

"Yeah, but look what happened with Cantor. You think those guys didn't know what they were up to?" asked Tyrell.

"Which guys? The Chinese or the manufacturer?" asked Kat.

"Well, those Chinese knew for sure. But the big guys were looking out for their bonus checks, using dirt cheap labor in China," said Lonny.

"Yeah, and those frat boys in the white house protect 'em," added Tyrell.

Well, Lonny and Tyrell certainly found something they have in common, though Kat had to warn them again about making up their minds before the evidence was all in. After dinner and more heated discussion, they broke up for the night, agreeing to meet up again at six a.m. sharp.

Kat did not have her usual trouble of falling asleep in the room, thanks in part to three glasses of mediocre wine that had pushed away the images of the victims in the MedWatch reports. She drifted off to sleep with one last hope: that the work that would begin tomorrow would go well.

The three pulled into the NorthAmerican-Genberg parking lot in a caravan, flashing their identification to get by security to pull into spaces right in the front of the lot. They hustled into the building before security could alert too many departments, identified themselves and let the receptionist know that the company had thirty minutes to allow them access to the facilities before NorthAmerican-Genberg would be accused of blocking an investigation. The poor girl looked terrified and frantically called every extension she could think of to try to get someone in charge down to the lobby ASAP. Kat knew it was early, earlier than most suits bothered to get to work, but that wasn't her problem. She couldn't have cared less whether they had to get someone there in their pajamas. She just wanted immediate access to the facility and was throwing around all the weight she had.

"Good morning, Miss Vasquez!" said the very perky blond who strode in through the front door to greet her. She must have been dispatched from the nearby corporate offices.

"I'm Pamela Connolly, from the Media depart—" she began.

"We're not interested in PR. Someone from operations needs to get here. Fast." Kat cut in.

"We've contacted all of our top people, and someone should—"

"You've got fifteen minutes to produce someone who can get us access to the entire facility. In the meantime, we're not interested in talking to anyone else," Kat said flatly.

The poor girl looked like she was going to cry before scampering down the hallway, presumably to go find someone, anyone, who had finally gotten to work. Kat felt bad for her, but whoever put her on the firing line should have known better. Another fifteen minutes passed before a distinguished looking, middle-aged man appeared to greet them. He was Fred Myers, VP Operations for the location. Kat showed him the inspection paperwork and he led them into the facility where they split up for their various assignments. Tyrell was escorted by one employee and Lonny another. Myers personally led Kat into an office where the appropriate paperwork awaited her, promising to have Tyrell and Lonny returned to her at the end of their inspections.

She spied the piles of reports and logbooks and sighed, wishing for a cup of coffee to help her through the review. Almost as if on cue, a young woman who identified herself as Myers' assistant appeared with two cups of coffee, one regular, one decaffeinated, and a pot of hot water, in case tea was her preference. Kat gratefully accepted the cup of regular and the girl left, promising to return in a couple of hours to collect another beverage request.

She plunged into the financials first, leaving the logs for Tyrell and Lonny later. She concentrated on NorthAmerican-Genberg's biggest clients, analyzing orders and delivery schedules and comparing them to MedWatch reports. This was the informational stage of the investigation, so as she surveyed reports, she marked where important data was so she could refer to it later in preparing her spreadsheets. Mostly, Kat tried not to draw any conclusions yet. Early judgments translated into the very real possibility that something would get missed later on. Hastening to "expose" a problem was as dangerous as the FDA's policy of fast tracking, hastening to grant approval to drugs that haven't yet undergone thorough independent testing and trials.

As promised, Myers' assistant reappeared two hours later, time which seemed to have moved far more quickly for Kat. The first cup of coffee had hit her bladder probably an hour ago but Kat was just now aware of it again. The assistant kindly led her to the ladies' room, then continued down the hallway to retrieve another beverage for Kat—this time, a Diet Pepsi. Myers' assistant was waiting for Kat in the office when she returned, a soda can in one hand and a sheaf of menus in the other.

"Mr. Myers wanted me to ask you if you wanted any lunch brought in," said the young woman.

Kat was surprised at how hungry she was, and then was even more surprised at her answer to the young woman.

"I would really like a real Philadelphia Italian hoagie," she announced.

The girl's face lightened up and she immediately pulled out the appropriate menu from her pile.

"You want a real Italian hoagie, or a New Jersey Italian hoagie?" the girl asked while holding back the menu as though Kat had to earn a glance at it.

"Capicola, prosciutto, mortadella, good provolone, oregano, and oil. Oh, and sweets on the side. But especially the roll, Sarcone's if possible. Amoroso's, if necessary," Kat said clearly pleasing the girl.

"This place makes the best," she declared, handing the menu for Angelo's to Kat.

Kat surveyed the typical pizza place take out menu, then called Lonny and Tyrell to see if they wanted anything, but both decided to continue their on-sites and break for an early dinner instead. Kat confirmed her order to the girl, who then exited the room. Kat knew from experience that the way to gain trust in the Philadelphia area was to appreciate the quirks of the food scene. She didn't know whether Myers was a native of the area or not, but if he was, the message of her order would buy her some mileage with the guy.

While she waited for her lunch, Kat continued to go over documents and set aside a pile that she would request copies of to review back at the hotel. So far, she hadn't seen anything overtly suspicious, but then, she hadn't imagined that she would. This kind of operation would take some digging to find. What she also knew was that time was not on her side. People were already sick and there were hundreds of deaths. She knew there might be another casualty for every minute wasted. She grabbed her cell as it buzzed its way across the table and answered it before checking the caller ID.

"Change of plans. I'm not coming into town tomorrow," said Jimmy, oblivious to the fact that Kat wasn't at home anyway.

"Too busy or crisis?" Kat asked more to make conversation than anything else. "Emergency summit at Jefferson," he replied.

Kat frowned and stared at the wall in front of her as his words sunk in. "What's that about?" she finally asked.

"I don't have to tell you guys that there've been a lot of MedWatch reports lately," he said.

Kat clutched. Had someone leaked out some details from the investigation or was this coincidence?

"This just Jefferson, or citywide?" she asked, trying to sound casual.

"Far as I know, it started as just Jeff, then politicians got involved. What do you guys know?" he asked.

Jimmy knew full well that she could not answer that question for him and for a moment the thought crossed her mind that he was inappropriately probing for information, rather than just innocently making conversation with a friend. She had to play this carefully though, because he did call her with the tip on Jefferson.

"Jimmy, listen—" she began.

"Hey, nothing serious, right?" he interrupted.

Kat wasn't sure whether he was referring to the present conversation or to their relationship, but she chose not to respond either way.

"This thing at Jefferson public?" she asked.

"Far as I know. Listen, got a meeting. See you soon?" he asked.

Kat hung up without answering. If Jimmy was correct about the Thomas Jefferson University Hospitals summit, that meant this thing was about to break in the press and that meant however quickly her team was working, it wasn't fast enough. Now the distributors, including whoever was behind the counterfeits, were going to be on the lookout for the FDA and even more underground in their activities. She knew this would have happened eventually, but she was hoping for at least another week before the lid was off of this story. She clicked the Dan's speed dial on her phone.

"What's up Kat?" asked Dan.

"You heard about this 'summit' at Jefferson tomorrow?" she asked.

"First I'm hearing of it. What do you know?" he asked.

"Just heard from one of my distributors that it's happening, but that's all I know so far," she replied.

"That's gotta be Conroy," Dan said, referring to Senator Patrick Conroy, longest sitting US Senator from Pennsylvania.

"I hope it's not public," Kat said, tapping her pen on the table.

"Maybe page six type stuff at this point. But something like that could push it to page one," Dan replied.

"I know. Anybody else on the story?" Kat asked, dreading the answer.

"Regular beat guys sniffing around, but all they've got is the public reports. They're not working too hard on it at this point, but with a little more detail they might get really interested. Sounds like you need to be there tomorrow," he said.

"Right. I just don't… you know I can't work under a microscope," she replied, hoping Dan would catch the drift of her statement and keep the department quiet.

"We're not answering questions out of here. And I'm going to keep it that way," he confirmed.

Kat was grateful for the department's tight-lipped policy. It meant that she could go to Jefferson tomorrow as a concerned party and not an FDA investigator. The last thing Kat wanted to do was be party to a Senator trying to make a name for himself by capitalizing on a serious situation.

"Thanks Dan."

"Oh, Kat. Don't want to rush you but things seem to be progressing pretty quickly out there. I don't know how much longer I can keep this under wraps."

Dan's message was loud and clear: Kat and the rest of the investigators needed to come up with something soon, before the lid got blown off the story and everyone closed ranks. Whoever was behind what was happening was going to be driven underground, making them even harder to find. Kat just hoped that the trail of lot test results led them somewhere soon.

Lonny and Tyrell finished around five o'clock and Kat sent them back to the hotel, since they had worked through lunch. She stayed and pored over financials for a few more hours. She would have stayed longer, but she felt sorry for Myers and his assistant who were stuck there as long as she was on-site. She left with a pile of papers and some logbooks to review back at the hotel, fantasizing that she might be able to work in a steamy hot tub.

As she passed the hotel bar, Kat heard snippets of what sounded like a heated discussion between two men and quickly recognized Lonny and Tyrell's voices. She sighed heavily and hung her head before peeking back into the bar. The two of them were head to head.

"So, my man, Stokley Carmichael was the real hero!" said Tyrell.

"There's no Stokley Carmichael day," Lonny answered.

"That's just it! That's what I saying about how whites picked black heroes—" began Tyrell.

Kat rolled her eyes and made a beeline toward them. The last thing she needed tonight was to play referee.

"Hey guys, how's it going?" she interrupted.

"Heeey, Miss Kat. Lemme get you a drink. Bartender, one Pinot red here," called Tyrell.

"Little wound up, huh Tyrell?" Kat half joked. She sat down at their table.

"Just blowing off some steam. Just blowing off steam."

Kat looked at Lonny's face to see if his expression matched Tyrell's assessment.

"Tough day," Lonny said raising his glass, clinking his ice cubes.

The waiter dropped off Kat's glass of wine and she took a sip before continuing. Just her presence seemed to settle the two down and Kat hoped that was enough to send the message to the two of them that they needed to watch themselves. She understood the need to blow off steam, but under the circumstances, they needed to be as inconspicuous as possible.

"Anything today?" she finally asked of them both.

"Nothing obvious," answered Lonny.

"Looked good where I was today. Have to wait for the sample test results," said Tyrell.

"I think things are heating up, so we've got to move faster than we thought," said Kat.

"Ah, you heard about the Jefferson thing tomorrow," asked Tyrell.

"What did you hear?" Kat asked.

"Overheard a QA person while I was on-site. Told my friend Lonny here--" answered Tyrell.

"I called up couple of good ole paper boys, friends of mine, and they're all over the story," added Lonny.

"Here or in WV?" asked Kat.

"Both. Press is catching wind of something going on," said Lonny.

"Shit! Then this is going to be out tomorrow," said Kat.

Lonny said, "Oh, Senator Conroy's going to make it come out tomorrow, just in time for the evening news."

Kat stared absently at the both of them while she ran the scenarios through her brain. She needed to be at the summit, but she had to make sure that Conroy wasn't aware of how much presence the FDA had in the area or how big the problem had become.

"You gotta go, right?" asked Tyrell.

"Have to," she replied. "Can't be in the dark about what's being said. I already talked to Dan and the department's keeping their mouth shut.

"Don't know how long they can keep that up," said Lonny. "Hey, listen, Lonny and me here, we're good. We're veeeerrry good. We will move through that place tomorrow like fire."

"Sounded a little less than good, just now, Tyrell," Kat said.

"No, no, see we were just talking history here. White folks history and black folks history, you know?" said Tyrell.

Kat looked at Lonny again for confirmation. The last thing she needed was any kind of tension between these two.

"I'm enjoying Tyrell's education," said Lonny.

"Don't you worry 'bout a thing. We're gonna be back at NorthAmerican-Genberg tomorrow and be ready with something or to hit the next site. Right my man?" Tyrell slapped Lonny on the shoulder.

Lonny laughed, bumping fists with Tyrell. Kat had to keep from laughing.

She finished her glass of wine and bid goodnight to the guys, reassured that they could handle the rest of the inspections. She went upstairs to check on the rest of her crew.

It had been a long first day, the first of many to come, and Kat as no closer to solving this crime than she was a day earlier. She knew it was unreasonable to assume that anything would have turned up so quickly, but it still didn't prevent her from hoping. She thought of all the families of victims and patients like Jorge who were in danger and wished that she could have immediate answers for them. She checked the department website to see whether any additional reports were logged and to her dismay, found another fifty MedWatch reports added in one day. Now she wished she had stopped and bought a bottle of wine on her way to the hotel, because she was going to need it all in order to some sleep. Those fifty new reports would haunt her dreams. Not just words on a page, but real people suffering, maybe even dying. The 27-year old bone marrow transplant patient living with dangerous and uncontrolled rejection because of a substandard dose of immunosupressants; the 54-year old heart patient unable to care for her three foster kids because her antidysrhythmic meds were substandard; the babies sickened from poisonous counterfeit vaccines… And she wasn't sure why yet. It was only a matter of time before there were more deaths—and time was running out.

***

Colton headed to his condo to get ready for his big evening with Cherie. He planned to propose over dinner, and then take her to Club Rouge, where sixty of their friends were waiting to surprise them with an engagement bash. Langford and Patricia would be there, of course, and Colton fantasized about the jealous look on Langford's face when he saw Cherie's ring. His old college roommate, Mr. Main Line Money, Mr. Philadelphia Society, partner in daddy's law firm, would have to admit to himself that Colton Barnes was giving him a run for his money.

Since the day they had first met, Langford lorded his money and status over Colton. During their Penn days, Langford invited him on trips or to parties at the family's house in the Hamptons, where Colton was no longer on even footing with Langford. It wasn't always *what* Langford said, but *how* he said it, how he smugly spoke of those with less, how he expected the world to lay down at his feet, and how he considered himself one of the country's elite that grated on Colton. Although Colton had enjoyed many of the same trappings as Langford—the private school, the Ivy League education, the trust fund—it was clear that Colton was never really a member of the club, nor would he ever be. Even the rich had their hierarchy and how old the money was and how it was made was what mattered. Daddy Barnes grew up piss poor in Texas and made his money as a football coach and sports commentator. It didn't take Colton long to realize that his father was invited to parties for the novelty and for bragging rights, but that no one was seriously interested in making a lifelong friend with him. He hated that his father was too naïve or too stupid to realize that, and he hated even more having to go places with his father where he was clearly out of his league.

The difference between him and his father was that he was educated and a business owner, not just some performing clown. He might still be one of the nouveau riche, but he knew how to cultivate the proper habits of the rich and exploit them for his own benefit. Marrying Cherie was a stroke of genius, another step in achieving his goal. The fact that he actually happened to like her was a bonus.

Colton lingered in the bathroom, contemplating whether Cherie's thrill at the proposal and the ring alone would be enough to insure a great screw afterwards or whether he should take one of his stash of little blue pills. Then he remembered that Patricia would be there and how just being around her could make him hard.

As he finishing shaving, Cherie came home from work and plopped on the bed. She looked tired and he was immediately irritated. He didn't want anything to interfere with his perfect evening.

"Rough day?" he asked, trying to hide his irritation.

"I'll be fine. I just need a few minutes off my feet."

He wiped off his face and lay down next to her on the bed. He stroked her hair and hoped to get her to feel better quickly because he didn't want to be late to the restaurant. She smiled at him and closed her eyes for a moment. Then seemingly energized from her short rest, she got up and headed to the bathroom.

Colton dressed in his new shirt and suit and admired himself in the mirror. He felt better about how the suit jacket hid his expanding paunch. He poured himself a Scotch, and then sat down on the bedroom chair to watch Cherie get ready.

She emerged from the shower not quite dry, caressing herself with the towel to banish the beads of water that clung to her silken skin. She tossed the towel in the laundry and stood naked, repeatedly running her fingers through her wet hair until she was ready to dry it. Her breasts gently bounced as she worked on her hair; it reminded him of how they looked when she was on top. He loved the way she left only a narrow strip of pubic hair in place and removed the rest, allowing him to glimpse a bit of her clit from between her bare lips. He didn't often want to kiss her there, but the sight of her like this made him think that he might allow his lips to explore her there later.

She stopped fooling with her hair and began to massage herself with lotion, beginning with her face and systematically making her way down her lovely body. He imagined his hands to be hers and felt himself stir at the memory of her soft, perfect skin. Then he caught a glimpse of her lovely cunt when she propped one foot up on the side of the toilet to examine her feet and check her toenail polish.

She smiled at him as she came into the bedroom and began to dress, fully aware that he watched her. He liked to see the panties and bra she chose, wanted to think about them all evening, next to her body, scented like her. He rarely spoke when he watched her and she learned that he wasn't interested in any conversation. He just liked to watch. The quiet heightened his excitement, left him with his own narration, and allowed him to think words he would not utter.

She chose a beautiful silk print halter dress, one that would cling nicely to her breasts and barely brush against her nice, rounded rump as she walked. His hand would be able to feel the exquisite softness of the silk as well as brush against her curves. Perhaps even Langford would catch a glimpse of his hand on her ass and imagine what he could not have.

"This okay?" she asked, breaking the silence.

"Nice," he replied, finishing the last drop of his Scotch.

"Do I have time for a drink?" she asked, slipping on her heels.

He checked the clock on the bureau. They had almost forty-five minutes until the driver arrived. Plenty of time for a drink but not enough time for a spontaneous fuck.

"I'll get it for you," he said, heading for the bar.

He poured himself another Scotch and a glass of chardonnay for her, and met her back in the bathroom where she was getting ready to work on her hair. Colton dropped off her drink and retreated to the living room where he snapped on the television to catch the last few minutes of the network news. He caught the tail end of a story about a Palestinian man who was helping to revitalize his neighborhood that had been bombed out in the latest Israeli attack and recognized the old man as the one with the necklace in St. Bart's. The Palestinian never revealed in the interview where he got the money to rebuild, he only spoke of how the Palestinians were a strong and determined people, a people who would never disappear. At first Colton was angry that his money was being used for mundane things, preferring to imagine that fighters of great courage used it to buy weapons, ammunition, and bomb making supplies. But as he watched the report, he found the old Palestinian endearing and even intriguing. He wanted to learn more about this man, spend time learning about his life, and listening to his tales. It was the first time he had cared about any of the men who came to see him.

"That suit is exquisite," Cherie said, startling him. You look wonderful. Is it new?"

He snapped off the set and jumped to his feet, shaking off thoughts of the Palestinian.

"Luigi," he answered. He kissed her lightly for her compliments. He checked his pocket for the jewelry box, and led Cherie to the front door. The driver waited for them out front.

"We're walking to the Ritz, but we'll need you later," he said.

"Shall I expect a call from you Mr. Barnes or the valet?"

"Valet."

"Very good, sir."

"We're going somewhere after dinner?" Cherie asked.

Colton just smiled, taking Cherie's hand and steering her north on Broad Street toward City Hall. The Ritz-Carlton was formerly a bank building, an imposing presence in classic Greek style with massive marble columns flanking the entrance standing in the shadow of the city hall. Colton had met Philippe, the executive chef, years ago at a bar late one night and the two became fast friends. Since then, Colton frequented the Ritz and made it a point to recommend the restaurant to friends, telling them to make sure the chef knew they were there on his recommendation. His patronage paid off and soon Philippe began to have one of his staff deliver a new dish to Colton at the condo, just to get his opinion.

They were stopped at the next intersection when Cherie suddenly leaned over and placed a soft kiss on Colton's cheek. He did love her; she was good for him, she was the right choice, but he did really love her. He knew it was not the love he had for Badia… as soon as he allowed her name to cross his mind, the memories flooded in with a stabbing sensation in his heart. Everything with Badia fell into place so easily, the conversation, the humor, dreams and aspirations, the sex. For the only time in his life Colton felt as though this was someone he could happily live out the rest of his life. She had no family here, two brothers and some other extended family in Afghanistan and Colton wanted so much to make a family with her, for her. She insisted that her brothers meet him first.

"They must approve," she had said.

The brothers were coming to the States on business to stay for a couple of months. The perfect time to meet and become close. Colton arranged for the brothers to house sit for a friend, a house big enough for Badia to stay with them.

"This is Dabir and Ameer," Badia introduced them.

Dabir was the older brother, darker, heavier and calmer. Ameer was younger, seemingly many years younger—wiry and twitchy, always on edge. Colton had a harder time being with Ameer, whose nervousness made Colton nervous and a bit paranoid. The brothers were busy all the time, with numerous phone calls, meetings, quiet conversations. Badia seemed thrilled to see them at first, and then became more withdrawn the longer they stayed. Once Colton arrived to find her in tears and Dabir speaking at her with a raised voice and it took all his restraint not to pop Dabir in the face.

"No, no, you do not understand, my love," said Badia and she stood and hugged him.

"She wants to go pay her respects to the family of a lost friend and I will not let her," said Dabir.

Colton looked at Badia for confirmation. Her tears had left trails of eye makeup down her face, which she smeared with the back of her hand.

"He was a childhood friend of mine. We were as close as siblings, closer maybe. Taliban killed him," she said. More tears flowed and she clung to Colton. Her brothers scowled.

That was the last he saw of her. Now he kicked himself for letting her leave with her brothers, for letting her out of his sight. Although he vowed to search for her to the ends of the earth, Dabir made it clear that she was never to be found. Colton was lost for years, dead to the world and willing to help those who were also dead and wanted the world dead.

And now, he was about to ask Cherie to marry him. He had not believed in love since Badia. Before that he never believed in love if it was his parents' version of it—raging and humiliating, dismissive and self-serving. With Cherie, he felt the closest he had to what seemed like love again. He squeezed her hand a little and led her one more block to the Ritz-Carlton.

"Mr. Barnes!" Samuel the Maître d' said as they entered.

"Good to see you, Samuel."

"Ahhh, and this must be the beautiful Cherie."

Samuel reached out and gently took Cherie's hand, bringing it to his lips for a light kiss. Cherie blushed.

"We hope you have a wonderful evening with us." He led them to a table by the window with a view of the city. A bottle of chilled Cristal waited for them, which Samuel quickly opened and poured.

"What's the occasion?" Cherie asked, startled.

"First, a toast," Colton replied. He lifted his glass, tapped it with Cherie's, and took a sip.

"Okay, so…" she began.

"Then, this," he said.

Colton pulled out the ring box and opened it in front of Cherie. Then, without much of a pause, he rushed to propose.

"Will you be my wife?"

He watched her face as she glanced at the ring, and then quickly looked at him. The way she looked at him, long and deep, made him feel as though she had penetrated his soul. He had never felt that before. He had never allowed anyone to gaze at him that intently. He was startled by the thought that someone else understood his most intimate thoughts. He felt a bit light-headed and glad that he was still sitting in his seat instead of next to the table, down on one knee.

"Of course." She lightly touched the ring and smiled.

He slipped it on her finger, and surprised himself at how sweetly he kissed her afterward. Though he had calculated the entire event, it surprised him at how much he felt. He could hear muted "ahhs" and "ooohs" from other diners in the restaurant. He watched Cherie's smiling eyes. He took a drink of champagne and tried to relax. It shocked him that he felt so emotional. It made him nervous. His heart continued to beat hard and felt agitated, as though he were a caged animal. He regretted having done this in public and wished that he had just asked Cherie at home, alone.

"This was quite a surprise," she said.

He could barely hear her. When he looked up at her, her face looked different to him now, flushed and glowing, more excited than he had ever seen her. He found himself taking big swigs of his champagne and touching everything on the table in an effort to steady himself. Cherie spoke to him and he could see her speaking, but he didn't hear what she said. Only the background noise of the room registered in his head. Finally, he felt her hand on his and began to reconnect with her in the room. She hadn't seemed to notice his reaction. He tried to focus on ordering his dinner, but could not, so he flagged down the waiter and ordered a double Scotch. The smoky sting of the Scotch finally brought him fully back to himself. He drank another one just to make sure. During dinner Colton relished the sight of that perfect stone on Cherie's finger, mesmerized with each movement of her hand and how the ring caught the light. He was fixated on how jealous Langford would be, on how Langford would have to realize that Colton was on his level.

Philippe appeared from the kitchen with their coffee and brandy and a special dessert for two.

"Congratulations! When will the happy day be?" he asked.

Before Colton could even consider the question fully, Cherie jumped in with an answer.

"Next year. Planning takes at least a year," she replied.

"And I am sure when you are planning your wedding that you will consider having it here!" Philippe exclaimed.

"Absolutely." Cherie didn't hesitate.

Colton hadn't thought beyond tonight but now he realized that he would soon be in the thick of wedding planning on top of everything else he had to deal with. He squelched his instinct to groan and focused on getting to Club Rouge. He called the valet and had him alert his driver that they were ready to leave.

"Can I know where we're going now?" she asked as they were getting into the limo.

"I rented out Club Rouge," he replied.

"For just us?" she asked.

"And a few hundred family and friends."

Cherie gasped and squeezed his arm and Colton was proud that he made her happy. The club was only a couple of miles away from the restaurant but the ride was longer than usual, complicated by some police activity in the area. Colton used the time to slip his hand up Cherie's leg and retrieve some of her scent on his fingers, a scent he would enjoy as he sipped his drinks, a scent he would hold over all the other men at the club. She giggled as he waved his fingers in front of his nose and smirked.

The driver pulled up to the unassuming entrance to the club, and jumped out to open the limo door. Colton and Cherie entered the dark, smoky club and were greeted by a sudden surge of light and a spirited cheer of "Surprise!" Colton put his arm around her shoulder and hugged her tight. Then he raised his arms and let out a triumphant yell.

Jackie Jr. presented them each with a glass of champagne and the crowd raised their glasses in a toast. Colton surveyed the crowd for Langford and Patricia but first caught sight of his parents standing by the bar. Daddy looked about ten whiskeys into the night, red faced and slumping onto the bar to steady himself and as always, Mom stood by him, oblivious. Neither one of them were smiling. Colton hoped he could avoid them for the night. He continued to scan the room and finally found Langford and Patricia standing next to Langford's parents, Albert and Kitty. When they met his gaze, they raised their glasses in a toast and beamed. Colton felt like he had climbed to the top of the world. A hundred prominent Philadelphians and the important Wentworths were here for him and Daddy had to witness it, whether he liked it or not. He had looked forward to a moment like this the first time he felt one of his father's barbs. He had even dreamt about it, yet doubted that it would ever happen.

"It's about time! I thought my son would never ask this girl and she'd get away like every football he ever tried to catch," shouted his father from the other corner of the room.

The crowd laughed politely at Daddy Barnes. Colton narrowed his eyes. As angry as he was, he took solace in knowing that now he had superseded his father. He was now the alpha male; he was now the powerful Mr. Barnes.

"I would like to propose a toast," called out Langford.

The crowd hushed and waited for him to continue.

"To Colton and Cherie. May they be as happy as Patricia and me, and may they enjoy as many years of happiness as there are years to their lives," he said.

Langford raised his glass and the crowd followed suit. Colton clinked his glass with Cherie's and the two took a drink, and then Jackie motioned for the DJ to start the music. The room exploded with light and thumping, pulsating music that rattled the glasses at the bar and got the crowd moving in spite of themselves. Colton grabbed Cherie's hand and led her through the crowd of well-wishers and over to the Wentworths. "Thanks for the toast, buddy," he said to Langford, shaking his hand.

He watched as Langford leaned over and gave Cherie a kiss on each cheek, stealing a glimpse of her breasts down the front of her dress as he did. Colton had to contain his glee. He knew what Langford was thinking and it was exactly what he wanted Langford to think. Then Colton leaned over and gave Patricia a kiss on the cheek, "accidentally" brushing his hand across her breast as he leaned in. She seemed unaware of his hand and simply continued the conversation as though nothing out of the ordinary had happened. He checked to see whether Langford had seen what he had done, but Langford's gaze was still fixed on Cherie.

"You two look so happy!" Patricia gushed.

"We're so happy for you," added Langford.

"It's like watching my own son," said Albert, clapping Langford on the back. Patricia reached out and grabbed Cherie's hand to examine the ring, and as she did, Colton carefully watched Langford's face. He would never say a word, but he would know that things were not as they were before, that never again would Langford be able to discount Colton, never again be able to think of himself as superior.

"It's beautiful," remarked Kitty.

The six continued with their small talk, but Colton had grown bored and wanted a drink and to mingle around the party more. He knew better than to ever walk away from the Wentworths and so he stayed, struggling to pay attention to their annoying conversation.

"…at the club, and I was astonished at the…" yammered Kitty, while Albert mentioned something about golf and Palm Beach and Langford corrected Patricia about the divorce settlement between the Bidley heirs.

"Oh, you must come with us!" Patricia exclaimed.

"If Colton could get away," Cherie said, tapping his arm and bringing him back to the conversation.

"Ah—" Colton began, looking to Cherie for help.

"Langford and Patricia are going to the Palm Beach house next week and they asked whether we were interested," said Cherie.

"Sounds good. I'll have Betsy check," said Colton.

"It would be good to get out of the cold up here," said Patricia.

Colton watched as Langford seemed to lean in closer to Cherie with his eyes fixated on her breasts. Colton figured he was probably enjoying the idea of being in the same house as her for a few days. Though Colton had always lusted after Patricia and coveted her, now he had lost interest. Without any interest in Patricia, Colton had little interest in allowing Langford near Cherie. He knew he was too busy to go to Palm Beach for a week. He had to suffer through another dismal trip to China, and one to the plant in Manchester. But there was no point in revealing any of that to the Wentworths. Let them think he was coming and he would handle the decline later. He was about to excuse himself and make the rounds around the room when he caught a snippet of conversation between Langford and Albert that peaked his interest.

"FDA's crawling all over the manufacturers lately," said Langford.

"TemePhelps got any exposure?" asked Albert.

"Waiting for test results," answered Langford.

The music was loud and Colton had to lean over to hear what they were saying. Albert tapped him on the shoulder and asked, "Colton, you hearing anything from customers?"

"Nothing out of the ordinary, as far as I can tell," he lied.

He knew very well that he was receiving increasing complaints from locations that were seeing more allergic reactions, but he was able to produce verification that there were no issues at his facility. That successfully deflected fault to the manufacturer.

"Somebody's in panic mode at the FDA," answered Langford.

"Started with the Heparin thing," said Colton.

"They got that under control. Now they're in paranoia mode, rattling all cages, searching under all rocks," offered Albert.

"Overstepping?" Colton asked, a little worried.

"Not yet. Might be a matter of time," answered Langford.

"That's what we're there to prevent," added Albert.

Albert excused himself and went off to the bar with Kitty. Patricia and Cherie decided to follow. Langford and Colton were left alone.

"I'm surprised, I thought guys like TemePhelps had their own in-house counsel," said Colton.

"They do. But they're using us too, rather than ramp up their staff," answered Langford.

"Nice gig," Colton remarked.

"Good billable hours. Lot of headaches though. Pretty big learning curve," said Langford.

"Let me know if I can help out, explain anything to you guys."

He was pleased with how cool he played that last exchange, pleased also that Langford would take him up on his offer for advice. But, he was worried about hearing that the FDA might be on some kind of alert status. He made a mental note to alter his ratios to put more legitimate product on the market until things died down a bit. He would have to put out feelers to see how widespread the reports were and calculate what the past couple of weeks of product might mean to future reports. If the FDA had already started on the manufacturers, it was going to take some time for them to complete all the testing and draw some conclusions before they could take any action. Of course, they weren't going to find anything. Then they would have to move to the next step and that meant the wholesale distributors. He had to make sure all of his books were in order, that there was no "alternative" supply in the pipeline or on any of his premises. He was going to have to mobilize his guys, making sure they all were able to pass an interview and all scrutiny from investigators. He had been through routine inspections. The question was, how much had the FDA ramped up and what would an inspection be like now? He needed somebody close to the investigators, somebody who could get him information.

He tried to put business thoughts out of his head until tomorrow and instead made his way around the room, greeting, glad handing, and talking to his guests. He realized that an hour had passed and he hadn't seen Cherie. As he scanned the room in search of her, he spotted Jackie and Langford whooping it up like college frat boys. He pushed his way through the crowd to get to them.

"Here's the man of the hour now," said Langford. Both Jackie and Langford were laughing uncontrollably. Langford slung his arm over Colton's shoulder. They were closer to the huge sound system and Colton had to lean in to hear what they were saying.

"What?" he asked.

"We were just talking about the time…you fucked that fat chick—" Langford said.

"*Really* fat chick," Jackie added.

"…right in front of the window—" Langford continued.

Colton tossed Langford's arm off of his shoulder and said, "Yeah, because if you'd been on top of her, you'd never get near her with your tiny dick!"

"…and some girl… some girl in the building across from ours… posted the video on the Internet!" Langford finished.

"I think they called it jiggle, wiggle or something!" Jackie added.

"I wonder whether it's still up there," Langford said.

The two doubled over with laughter. Colton stood fuming, digging for something to say.

"That was like, what, only the second time you got laid all year?" said Jackie.

"Must have been one more time than you've been laid since you married that big mouth cunt," Colton leaned in and said in Jackie's ear.

Jackie reeled back from Colton and stopped laughing, Langford looked puzzled. Colton got close to Langford's ear and said, "And all you've been thinkin' about all night is how you'd like to fuck Cherie. But she doesn't like pencil dicks."

Like Jackie, Langford jerked back away from Colton. "Hey, c'mon man. Lighten up. It was a joke. We were just joking around," he said.

"I know. Hey, I was just having a few laughs too," Colton replied, laughing.

The two stood silently with scowls on their faces, trying not to make eye contact with Colton. He felt victorious that he had shut down their banter and tried not to smirk. Colton resumed scanning the room for Cherie and finally saw her near the door, talking to Albert and Kitty.

Colton hurried his way across the room and caught up with them just as they were putting on their coats.

"Leaving so soon?" he asked as he wrapped his arms around Cherie from behind. She leaned her head back on his shoulder.

"Oh, there you are! We wanted to say congratulations again before we left you two love birds," said Albert.

"We're looking forward to the wedding," sang Kitty.

Colton stepped away from Cherie, gave Kitty a hug and kiss goodbye and reached out to shake Albert's hand. Albert grabbed Colton's hand and pulled him toward him in a warm embrace, surprising Colton. Just then, Langford and Patricia appeared.

"Okay chump, nice party, but it's time for us to go," interrupted Langford.

Colton noticed Langford's annoyance and was secretly thrilled that he was there to witness Albert's hug and even more thrilled that it seemed to get under his skin. Albert held the door open for Kitty and the two of them left just as Langford and Patricia slipped on their coats.

"Thanks for stopping by," said Colton as he shook Langford's hand. Langford limply shook Colton's hand but avoided any eye contact. Colton gave Patricia a quick kiss goodbye while Langford barely hugged Cherie. With the two of them standing so close together, Colton could now clearly see how much prettier Cherie was than Patricia.

"Don't forget, if I can be of any help in that TemePhelps thing," Colton said as they stepped toward the door.

Langford didn't reply.

Chapter 7

Form FDA 3500A, Incident #196,876 - 197,011:

...One hundred and thirty-nine third grade students from Wilson Elementary School in Camden, N.J., became sick after receiving the tetanus toxoid vaccine booster. One child died. The tetanus vaccine is most commonly combined with diphtheria and acellular pertussis. Incidences of allergic reaction or side effects from the vaccine have been noted as less than 1 in 16,000, with most side effects attributed to the pertussis component of the vaccine. Allergic reactions to the tetanus vaccine are rare and fatalities are rarer still.

Some of the first recipients at Wilson Elementary complained of slight discomfort, were placed under observation, and did not present any additional symptoms. School and medical officials attributed initial symptoms to fear of needles. No additional reactions were noted and officials administered the vaccine to all 137 third grade students.

Hours after administering the vaccine, all 137 students showed signs of allergic reactions. Students presented with rash, fever, swelling, and difficulty breathing, which in one case progressed into anaphylactic shock and death.

Testing results revealed that the vaccines contained a host of deadly bacterial contaminants, including improperly conditioned tetanus toxin; that is, live tetanus bacteria. FDA was able to track down vaccine source in India and is still actively investigating the local supplier of the vaccines…

***

Kat braced herself as she read over the agenda and then scanned the auditorium to see who was there from the manufacturers and wholesalers. Those guys must be sweating. She wondered how many of their corporate lawyers were here. Almost every seat on the lower level of the auditorium was filled and the aisles were clogged with people trying to get to whatever seats remained. The spin doctors and damage control teams were on full patrol, handing out literature to the press and trying to scope out the physicians and administrators. It was clear from the list of speakers that this was a serious summit and not some PR stunt. All the national and local media were there, corralled in the center of the auditorium with the best views of the speakers and Senator Conroy. Kat groaned.

As soon as Jefferson Hospital CEO, Ken Richardson came up to the microphone, people scurried to find seats and shutters began to snap.

"As most of you already know, this summit is in response to recent reports of drug abnormalities throughout the Jefferson Health Organization and the community it serves. We have assembled a panel of professionals who will share their findings and their expertise."

He introduced Senator Conroy, who took the opportunity to vow that Congress would do everything in its power to make sure the FDA was doing its job and protecting the American people. Kat groaned again, knowing full well the guys like Conroy were part of the reason why the FDA couldn't do its job well. Kat was all too familiar with the Senior Senator from Pennsylvania, as was every member of the FDA. He had been in office for over thirty years and developed a keen sense of how to keep himself looking relevant and involved in the news. That didn't always translate into getting things done for his constituents, or the American people, but it always resulted in making him appear as one of the most powerful men in the nation. He was one of the first to cut funding for the FDA, yakking about how government needed to become smaller and business should police itself; at the same time, he was always the first to complain that the FDA wasn't doing enough to keep the nation's food and drug supply safe. Since Kat's first encounter with him at a Congressional hearing, she could hardly stand the sight of the guy, let alone his grating voice. He finally finished and Richardson introduced the first speaker.

It was clear after the first speaker that what Kat's gut had told her was worse than she had imagined. Speaker after speaker—the emergency room physician, the EMT, nurses, pharmacists, and other healthcare professionals—recounted their observations of the last several weeks. She listened intently at first and took copious notes, but the panic kept rising up in her as the scope of the problem sank in. Some testing was already in and proved the supposition of substandard or adulterated product, but if the anecdotal evidence proved out in the rest of the lab results, virtually every single category of drug was affected, in each of its forms: oral dosage, injectables, and intravenous infusion. The magnitude of the problem made her heart pound hard. Dan must already have had an inkling of the disaster before he called them all to HQ.

***

Colton met Jackie at the office just as the sun was rising. It was too early to be awake after last night and far too early to be handling business affairs. But after Jackie's phone call, Colton had some cleanup work to do.

"I got coffee," Jackie said as he met Colton at the front door of USA Distributors.

Colton unlocked the door, grabbed the offered coffee, and led the way to his office. He sat down behind his desk and slumped over his cup. Jackie plopped a copy of the *Philadelphia Inquirer* on his desk with a loud thud.

"Inky's got it too," he said.

"That the guy you talked to last night?" Colton asked.

"No. Don't know this guy."

"Who was the guy who called last night?"

"Rubano," Jackie replied with more than a hint of disgust.

Colton caught Jackie almost rolling his eyes, tossing out a name Jackie obviously thought he already knew. Colton sat back in his chair and narrowed his eyes.

"Who the hell—" he began.

"The one who set his hair on fire at the frat party…" Jackie offered.

Colton sat up straighter in his chair, squaring his shoulders at Jackie.

"You got somethin' else you wanna say here?" he barked.

"No, no," Jackie said adjusting his tone.

"Good," Colton said.

He sat back in his chair again and reached for the newspaper.

"Rubano's a medical reporter for NBC now," Jackie finished.

Colton looked up from the paper. "Shit. How much he got?"

"Pretty good amount. No names or places, but he's onto the story pretty good. Watch out for him," offered Jackie. Colton motioned for Jackie to sit.

"He called you himself?" asked Colton.

"Remembered that my dad had a drug wholesale business and was looking for a perspective on the story," said Jackie.

Colton unfolded the paper in front of him and saw the headline: "Tainted or Counterfeit? Growing number of drug abnormalities cause alarm." The article enumerated a number of cases where patients were harmed or died from suspect medications. A sidebar gave the details of today's Jefferson summit.

Colton smirked, relishing the article and the idea of himself as the puppet master. Between this article and the summit, he would have to pull the counterfeits from his supply, at least for the time being, and stop deliveries. He didn't even want to think about what that was going to do to his shipments of money. On the other hand, he kind of looked forward to a trip to St. Bart's just for the surf and sun, with no obligations for meetings.

"This Inky guy seems to have a lot of information. How much you think Rubano knows?" Colton asked.

"Nothing more than anyone else. Told him I didn't have anything for him."

Colton eyed Jackie closely. He didn't like the idea of Jackie talking to a reporter and he certainly didn't trust that he was cautious enough with his words. Jackie studied his coffee cup like it was a detailed map.

"He's gonna be back," Colton said.

"I know. I said I had some guys I could call for information for him," said Jackie.

"Some guys? You gonna call him back?" Colton shot.

Jackie tore his eyes away from his coffee cup and locked gaze with Colton, and then spoke as though he were speaking to a child, "Noooo, I'm gonna wait for him to call me. I'm gonna have something to say to him just to throw him off the track."

Colton sprang to his feet and slammed his hands on the desk. Jackie jumped but stayed in his seat.

"You said what?" Colton bellowed.

"I, ah, I told him to let me know if the FDA's on it. And, whether they've got the FBI and the locals on it with them. Figured we might as well use him too," stammered Jackie.

He had changed his tone but Colton was still irritated. He kept his stare on Jackie until he shrunk down in his seat.

"I'm going to Jefferson," Colton suddenly said as he stepped around the desk. He had no interest in hearing the sob stories but he needed to see the faces and learn the names that might be out to hurt his enterprise. Much as he hated to admit it, his father had given him one good piece of advice over the years: know your opponent.

"What do you need me to do today?" asked Jackie.

"Start ramping up the legit orders; get enough supply in the warehouses to match the books. But, not too fast. Don't draw any suspicion. Use one of the subsidiary names if you have to. And make sure the guys in Jersey know that we're goin' legit. No mistakes now," Colton barked.

"Gonna be tough to get supply. Manufacturers are gonna make sure quarantines are done," Jackie said.

"Just get it done right. Can you handle that for once, Jackie?" said Colton.

He could tell by Jackie's face that he was annoyed, but it was designed to make sure Jackie didn't screw up.

"Been in the business longer than you, Colton," Jackie mumbled.

"You really just say that?" Colton demanded as he stepped closer to Jackie.

"Listen, I called you in on this, didn't I? Give me some credit for once," Jackie said. With that, he stood up and stepped closer to Colton.

Colton took a good look back at Jackie, assessing the reason for the defiance and considering how to punish him for it. Jackie, who normally squirmed under scrutiny, held himself firm. Maybe he would pop Jackie a good one in the face, but he remembered how tired he was from last night. Something was giving Jackie a backbone today. Colton made a note of it for the future.

"Just don't fuck up," Colton growled.

Jackie left the office without uttering another word, leaving Colton standing alone. He paced the room, tossed papers around his desk, and finally flung the newspaper across the room and swung at the air. He needed something to calm him down; things were getting too heated out there to lose his head. He needed something to make him feel better and he knew what always worked: attention to detail. The more he worked the details of his operation, the more he reassured himself that he could withstand any scrutiny. He sat down at his desk again, dug in his drawer, pulled out his personal laptop, and powered up. If local attention was on prescription meds, it was only a matter of time before this thing blew open nationally, and the FDA would be crawling over every facility. From the very beginning, he had kept an alternative set of financials on a completely separate computer, known only to Hugh and himself. Not even Nancy Wilcox, his CFO, knew about the second set. If the FDA did inspect the place, all they would see were the legitimate books and he had no reason to worry about not trusting anyone with his secret. Colton smirked at his own cleverness.

He retrieved the paper and scanned the article, looking for a time frame. According to the *Inquirer*, the first allergic reactions and other abnormalities were reported six weeks ago. He double-checked the spreadsheets to make sure it was the same time he starting ramping up his counterfeit ratio, suspicious that the Chinese were masquerading as a manufacturer and moving product directly themselves. Colton's blood pressure rose at the thought that some greedy Chinese were ruining his fastidiously laid plans.

He spent years doing his due diligence, calculating the average ratio per type of drug: one-quarter for drugs where symptoms would become obvious more quickly, one-half for drugs where they would not. He figured out the ratios drug by drug, and then studied MedWatch reports, adjusting for every blip that might make his endeavor detectible. If the counterfeits were thoroughly mixed in with the legitimate drugs, patients would get no more than a fifty-fifty split in a bottle, and usually less, for most drugs not enough to cause a detectable problem. He had an elaborate set of formulas for injectables too. It would take an unusual allergic reaction or a large number of reactions for the FDA to consider MedWatch reports worth an inspection. For the most part, he had designed the perfect business model. The FDA only had enough inspectors to show up about once every decade or so, so the odds were slim that he'd ever see them. Even if a drug did require an FDA inspection, the time frame was about six to eight weeks between a reported problem and when someone might come through the door. By that time he would have already remixed his shipments and gotten rid of any evidence of counterfeits. Now, it looked like someone was moving straight counterfeits into the marketplace, bringing far too much scrutiny to the business.

Colton stared at his computer screen, committing shipment numbers and ratios to memory so he could test them against the time frame and statistics that would certainly be quoted at the Jefferson summit. The more he studied, the angrier he got. His plan had been perfect and it still looked perfect on the screen in front of him. Those MedWatch reports were not his. They couldn't have been his. It had to be another player and he needed to find out exactly who. He packed up his laptop and headed out to Jefferson.

Traffic from the suburbs was light until he got close to Jefferson, where a fleet of press vans lined the narrow streets, clogging up traffic. As he squeezed past to the parking garage on 10th and Sansom, he saw the local affiliates and then the national press corps. He was contemplating the ramifications of national exposure when Cherie called on the cell.

"Don't forget our appointment at four o'clock today," she said.

"What appointment?" he asked.

"Don't tell me you already forgot," she countered.

"I don't have time for games, Cherie," he barked. Just tell me what the fuck you're talking about!"

"Are you okay?"

"I'd be better if you'd just tell me what you want," he said.

"We have a four o'clock appointment with the wedding planner today." She spoke so quietly he could hardly hear her.

"Jesus, Cherie. It's only been hours since the engagement. What's the big rush?" he sniffed.

"Colton, you forget what I do for a living. I know how much time these things take, and if we're aiming for next year, we've got to get working now," she countered.

He was silent while he parked the car and cut off the engine.

"Not sure whether I can get there on time," he replied evenly.

"Oh. Ah, I suppose I can take the first meeting myself and we can catch up later." She finished up with a long sigh.

He knew not appeasing her now would result in future complications. This was a new Cherie, emboldened by the ring, he guessed, one he was not used to dealing with. What would things be like after they married? This thought made him want to forestall the ceremony as long as possible. He got out of the car and walked toward the exit.

"Where is it? I might be able to make it if it's not too far," he offered.

"I set it up for our condo, but I can move it anywhere you want," she replied.

The Jefferson summit was likely an all-day affair, but the condo was only about a mile from where he parked. It was quite possible he could make it back in time. If he wanted to. He was sure he didn't want to be there for the meeting, or any of the other meetings regarding the wedding, and now he had to calculate how much he could miss and what the consequences would be.

"I should be able to get there late, depending on traffic," he finally said.

"I'd be so happy if you were here," she bubbled.

He hung up the phone and sighed, dreading however many months of this nonsense he would have to endure. He seriously considered proposing they fly some of their friends to some exotic location and just get it over with quickly. But he knew that, for Cherie, the event had to be in Philadelphia and it had to be covered by the local press. Besides, he had to admit that a lavish wedding would impress Langford and Patricia.

Just for a moment he chuckled when he thought of Cherie's Lancaster County country bumpkin parents in the middle of their daughter's Philadelphia society wedding. Tall and lanky Mr. Fulton, awkward and odd in his rented tux, and the enormous Mrs. Fulton stuffed into some sparkling mess of what she considered fashion. Then he couldn't help but think of his own parents and how his father would grandstand and spew a steady stream of derogatory comments until he passed out drunk or someone coaxed him out of the reception and into a waiting car. His mother would try her best to fix the situation, using up all the excuses she could conger up. Daddy's antics would likely make the local gossip column the next day; someone might even snap a picture. Colton sincerely wished the man would drop dead before the wedding.

Agitated even more now, Colton checked his watch, and then walked down Sansom Street to Jefferson. He entered the auditorium and took a seat near the back so he could survey the attendees. They must have expected a capacity crowd, because every single seat had a folder of information on it. Colton opened his and began to read the agenda, entitled, "Thomas Jefferson University Health System Summit on Drug Abnormalities."

Colton read the names and credentials of each speaker, feeling his beads of sweat begin to form on his forehead. While he expected the community members, the inclusion of specialists and researchers caught him off guard. Health care guys had been aware of this problem for more time than he'd assumed. There were already lab results and those took weeks. Had someone else moved into his territory or did his people in Jersey not follow directions? Now there were beads of sweat on his brow and lip.

"Colton Barnes, right?" said a skinny guy with stylishly ugly glasses who appeared at the end of his row of seats.

"Who wants to know?" Colton asked without looking up from his paperwork.

"You probably don't remember me, but I went to Penn with you and Jackie DeAngelo. Rob Rubano."

The guy held out his hand for Colton to shake. Colton looked the guy up and down, briefly regarding the khaki pants, the rumpled polo shirt and the digital recorder, and then shook his hand. He remembered how Jackie warned him to be cautious around the guy, but he also knew that if he could handle the terrorists of the world, he could handle some sniveling little reporter.

"You're the asshole who set his hair on fire, huh?" Colton said.

Rubano looked sheepish and Colton was proud that he was able to lay him out fairly quickly.

"Jackie says you and he are in business together. I guess you heard I talked to him," Rubano replied.

"And?" asked Colton.

"Just thought maybe I could use you guys as a resource, you know, opinions on what's going on with the drugs, what you're seeing on your end of the business. Background stuff," he replied.

"Jackie can fill you in. I'm really too busy myself," said Colton.

He turned back to the summit paperwork.

"Sure. I understand," said Rubano.

Colton hoped the conversation was over at that point and waited for the guy to leave, but instead he sat down next to him.

"So, how's your dad? Man, I still think Daddy was one of the best coaches in all the NFL," Rubano began.

Colton didn't feel the need to add to the conversation, and certainly had no interest in talking about his father. Silence settled between them until Rubano piped up again.

"Jackie told me he's married with a few kids. How about you? Married? Single?" he probed.

"How long you been working for NBC?" Colton knew this type of guy, who was really mostly interested in talking about himself and only asked personal questions so he could answer them about himself.

"I did an internship in my senior year and they hired me straight away. Worked the back room for a few years, but then got the chance to get on air and, you know, clicked with the public. I'm based out of New York…"

Colton turned off Rubano's noise and concentrated on scanning the faces in the crowd. The place was filling up rapidly. He ran over the list of speakers and recognized some of the specialists, the ones interviewed on the local news.

"… right?" Rubano suddenly finished.

"Looks like the press corps are over there," Colton pointed.

Rubano bolted out of his seat and took off, leaving Colton at peace.

***

In the middle of the infectious disease specialists' presentation on the increased occurrence of resistant strains of bacteria and super bugs, a commotion broke out in the back of the room. Kat couldn't see through the crowd, but a woman's voice clearly rose above the din.

"You killed my baby!" she screamed, and then somehow broke through the crowd and ran toward the dais, chased by a security guard and a few men from the audience. It was hard to tell the woman's age, she looked older than she dressed and dressed for a body that left her long ago.

"Murderers! Monsters!"

When she made it to the dais, she picked up a pitcher of water and dumped it on the person closest to her, an aide to Senator Conroy. One security guard managed to get his arms around the woman and began dragging her out of the room. Senator Conroy took the microphone.

"No, wait! Stop! Let her speak!"

The security guard stopped and let go of the woman, but continued to stand next to her in front of the dais. The crowd fell silent and all that could be heard was the racket of press cameras snapping shot after shot of the spectacle. Conroy stood firm at the microphone, glancing to make sure the press had their cameras aimed at him before he began speaking again.

"Ma'am. Can you tell us your name and what you've come to say?" asked Conroy.

He motioned her toward the microphone. Before the woman stepped forward, she straightened out her clothing and smoothed down her hair. The crowd patiently waited.

Now Conroy reached out to the woman, cutting a grandfatherly pose, pasting a look of sympathy on his wrinkled face. Kat cringed, dreading what was to follow.

Conroy motioned for security to retreat and again beckoned the woman to join him. She hesitated, so he came to her, put an arm around her shoulder and walked with her to the microphone. Whatever boldness she possessed when she crashed into the room had now left her and she stood, timid and silent at the microphone. Conroy took advantage of the silence, grabbed the microphone and introduced her.

"Ladies and gentlemen, this woman has a tale to tell and I think we need to give her the chance to speak. She may embody the anguish we are all feeling over this breach in our personal security."

He gently took the woman by the elbow and encouraged her to speak into the microphone. Her face still held the grimace of her rough entrance, though she softened the edges of it once she turned to see the faces staring back at her, waiting for her to speak. She leaned into the microphone and began.

"I'm… ah… I'm … my name is Diadera Witherspoon. My son Ray…" and those were all the words that came before she broke down in tears. Senator Conroy patted her back until she was able to continue. "My son is dead. He got the diabetes, and he needed his shots. Every day, two times a day he got the shots and he did good. Doctor said he doin' good, real good. He done good for three years, and then he gets kind of little red bumps all over, some kind of rash. I ask if he wants me to take him to the doctor, but he says, 'No Mom, they sprayed the fields at school where we have football practice, that's all' and I believe him… I believe him and I don't call the doctor." Here she broke down again and cried, but this time Conroy looked a little bored and stayed still, waiting for her to finally finish. "At night he takes his second shot like always and then he says he don't feel good. Then he's got this bad rash, really bad, and he starts like he can't breathe…I call for the ambulance. Lord, it was like about forever before they got there. He was not breathin' real good. I think his lips were blue. By the time they got there, he had passed." She sobbed quietly to herself. The room was silent.

Kat's mind raced through her memory, pulling up the one MedWatch report she read on an allergic reaction to insulin. The report stuck with Kat specifically, since allergic reactions to insulin had been rare for over a decade, once production moved from being isolated from pig pancreas to genetically engineered human insulin. In fact, the instance was so rare that even one case would be cause for alarm. This woman's son was not only a second case of allergic reaction, but also one that resulted in a death.

Kat jotted down notes on her papers about instructions for Lonny and Tyrell and research she needed stat from Maryanne. Her hand shook as she wrote.

"Thank you, Mrs. Witherspoon," said Senator Conroy as he motioned for someone to attend to her, and then retreated to his seat.

Kat had heard enough, but she didn't dare leave now. She was going to have to convince Dan that he needed to hold some kind of a press conference before these stories hit the national news.

"Little surprised to see you here," said Jimmy as he took a seat next to Kat.

Kat's heart jumped a little at the sight of him but she pushed down her emotion and put on her professional self.

"Why's that?" she asked.

"Figured you'd be out conducting an investigation or something."

"What makes you think we're not?"

"Conroy going to make it look like you guys are sitting around with your thumbs up your butts," said Jimmy.

"Can't do anything about that," she replied.

"Not so sure I'd want to be in the room once he gets started," he offered.

"Yeah, well. Goes along with the job I guess."

"You got guts, I'll hand you that. So, how long you in town for?"

Kat both couldn't and wouldn't answer the question. She didn't know how long she would be in town—maybe months after what she had heard today—and then again, maybe only a couple of weeks until Congress got its paws on these stories and called for hearings. She knew she needed a long talk with Dan.

"Don't know," she said.

"Good." He put his hand on her arm and smiled at her. She shifted in her seat, pulling her arm out from under his.

"For whom?" she asked.

"For both of us, I was hoping."

Kat tried not to pay attention to the twinge of excitement that shot through her and tried to ignore the hurt look on his face as she pulled her arm away.

"So, you've heard the evidence, Jimmy. What's going on?" She figured she'd turn the tables and see whether he could shed any light on the situation.

"Sloppy manufacturing or back door stuff out of foreign countries," he concluded.

"Hmmm. Maybe."

"Tell you what—let's have a discussion about this over dinner, shall we?" he asked.

"Jimmy, you know I can't—" she began.

"Why not?" he interrupted.

***

Colton enjoyed hearing the reports from the speakers. He relished how extensive his reach had become. He especially enjoyed the woman who charged up to the microphone and the drama she caused. Of course, he knew it was none of his doing, that it was either the work of the Chinese or junk from India. Insulin issues were too obvious and too risky, plus the profit margin wasn't worth the worry and he couldn't be bothered with the headache. What he did learn this morning was that someone was moving a great deal of product into the market indiscriminately and whoever it was would ruin things for everyone. Investigators would be crawling through everyone's business and the whole thing was just going to make it harder for everyone to operate. These guys had to be amateurs. Anybody in this game for the long term would have been more cautious. Whoever caused this mess was just looking to make a quick buck but they were taking it from the wrong person. The heat was on everyone now. Chances were these guys were now going to turn their attention to something safer, something the FDA wasn't likely to be eying up just yet. Cough syrup or children's pain relief syrups were likely targets—saturate that market and it would take years to be detected, if ever, and that was only if someone had an allergic reaction.

He couldn't control if these guys got a piece of his marketplace but his blood rose as he considered who the careless fuck was behind this. He made a mental note to tell Jackie to get the word out that he was holding a summit, laying down some ground rules and making it clear how to operate on his turf. In the meantime, he had to convert to a legitimate supply until the FDA was out of his hair.

The Senator called for a recess and Colton punched in Jackie's number.

"How's Jersey?" he asked.

"Fine. Got everything taken care of. They understand what's going on and we should be in new production as soon as tomorrow," he replied.

Colton snapped to his feet.

"Too soon!" he said too loudly, and then quieted down, suddenly aware of how many potentially dangerous ears could overhear him. He needed to set Jackie straight right now, before he did anything else stupid. He headed for the doors while talking. "You're risking running out of supply completely and that'll raise questions from customers! They know everything's short supplied for the time being. With what's going on, it's going to be that way for a while."

"Jesus Colton, have some faith in me, will ya? I made a few phone calls and managed to get some legit supply faster than anticipated, so we're good to go," Jackie replied.

Rubano was making his way over and Colton walked toward the nearest exit.

"Legit from where?"

"All over," Jackie said.

"All over, like from where?"

"India, China—"

"You gotta get domestic product or U.K., South American! Jesus, Jackie, haven't you been paying attention?"

Colton was suddenly aware that people were looking at him, more importantly that he may have caught Rubano's eye and ear. He rushed out of the hall as quickly as he could and found an empty hallway where he could scan both ways for anyone who might be listening.

"Colton, I know these guys. The product is good."

"Change it to U.K. or South American. Now!" he hissed, trying to keep his voice down.

"I don't—"

"Just do it!"

Jackie mumbled something about getting right on it, but by now Colton was so incensed that he could hardly hear Jackie's voice through the blood pounding in his ears. He paced the floor, slamming his heels into the carpet and moving up and down the hallway just trying to normalize his blood pressure.

"Listen, Jackie. We have to find out who these guys are. You hear me?"

"What guys?"

"Whoever's moving straight bad stuff. The reports are all over the place. These guys are careless and sloppy. We have to have a chat with them about that."

"I guess I could ask around…"

"Don't guess anything, just find out!"

Colton hung up his phone and shoved it into his pocket.

"Tough day, huh?" asked Rubano, who suddenly appeared over Colton's left shoulder.

Colton spun around and started to speak but quickly realized that opening up any kind of conversation with this guy was just dangerous. He just nodded and turned in another direction. Rubano followed him and now kept pace with him.

"So, what's your take on what's going on?"

"Going on where?"

"The summit."

For a moment, Colton was relieved to think that Rubano hadn't caught any of his exchange with Jackie and instead was focused on the summit.

"Lot of tragedies out there."

"So, what are you hearing from your customers?"

Colton was walking fast, just short of a sprint, hoping to shake Rubano, but the guy stayed with him. He burst through the doors to the auditorium and glanced around the room, desperate to find someone, anyone, to talk to. He spotted Jimmy on the other side of the room and made a beeline for him.

"Listen, man, I'd love to talk to you at some point, but right now I have some pressing business." With that, Colton waved at Rubano and left him standing near the door while he rushed to meet up with Jimmy.

***

"Good to see you again, Jimmy." Colton appeared unexpectedly next to Jimmy. Kat slumped in her seat and buried her head in the summit literature. The last thing she needed was the likes of Colton Barnes to make a note of her with Jimmy.

"Good to see you, Colton," she heard Jimmy reply.

There was a short silence, and then she felt a tap on her shoulder.

"Hi, Colton Barnes, USA Distributors. I saw you with Jimmy the other night at the Kammerly Center auction, right?" Colton held out his hand to shake.

"Kat," she said as she took his hand.

"Old friend from college, that right Jimmy?" Colton said.

Kat could tell from Colton's demeanor that he was quite pointedly engaging the two of them and Kat was trying to figure out why. She turned her back to him and pretended to answer a text message on her cell. She eavesdropped on his conversation with Jimmy and hoped that he would leave before she would have to speak to him again. Unfortunately, Colton sat down next to Jimmy and made himself comfortable. Kat gave up on the text messaging and picked up the summit materials again.

"So, Kat, what do you do that you're here today?" Colton asked.

"Concerned pharmacist," Kat lied.

"Philly area?" he asked.

"Maryland," she replied.

"You got your own independent or a franchise?" he probed.

"Don't try it Colton. She's a customer of mine," interjected Jimmy.

"Hey, gotta try at least, right Jimmy? So, what do you think about all this?"

Kat waited for Jimmy to answer.

"Kat? What's your take on all of this?" he repeated.

"Who knows?" she shrugged.

Though she wasn't interested in talking to him, she was fascinated watching Colton Barnes. Something about him struck her as just not right. He reminded her of the kind of frat boys she detested in college but there was more than that.

"I can't believe you don't have any thoughts on this," he persisted.

"Well, if there's anyone with answers, Kat's the one," Jimmy said, and then flashed a look that clearly showed how his mouth had gotten away from his brain.

"You got all the answers, huh?" Colton asked.

Kat made sure that Jimmy could see the annoyance on her face, and then tried to conger up an answer that would put an end to the conversation. She decided the best course was to excuse herself entirely.

"Listen, gotta go now. See you both around," She quickly took off toward the door.

She walked out as fast as she could and hoped that Jimmy didn't do anything stupid like try to follow her.

"What's her last name?" Colton asked.

"Vasquez," Jimmy answered.

"You makin' a move on her or what? 'Cuz if you're not, you're a fool."

Jimmy laughed.

"Why's that name familiar?" Colton mused. Jimmy tensed up at the question. So there was something about Kat that Jimmy needed to hide.

"Hey, congratulations! I heard you got engaged," said Jimmy.

"Word travels fast," Colton replied.

"Yeah, well, we travel in the same circles," said Jimmy.

"Do we, Jimmy?" Colton asked.

Jimmy looked a little startled by Colton's response, and cocked his head.

"So Jimmy, you ever talk to your partners about our conversation?" Colton began.

Now Jimmy sat up straight, taller than Colton.

"Haven't had the chance. We got a partner's meeting coming up and I'll float the idea then," said Jimmy.

"Dragging your feet on purpose?" Colton asked.

"No, like I said—" he began.

"Somebody else I should talk to instead?" Colton finished.

He wasn't really interested in making a move on Jimmy's company, but it was necessary to toss Jimmy around a bit.

"I said we have a partner's meeting coming up," Jimmy reiterated.

"I'm sure you and your partners are doing pretty well, huh?" Colton persisted.

"We're getting by," Jimmy answered.

"But see, you can do better than just getting by. A whole lot better. Better than you could have imagined. And if you help me with this deal, I could sweeten the pot for you, kind of like a sign-on bonus," Colton said.

"Colton, I really have to talk to my partners—"

"You ever been to St. Bart's, Jimmy? It's paradise. I've got a couple of villas down there. Maybe you and your Ms. Vasquez would like to fly down with me in the jet for a few days. Sound good?"

"I don't—" Jimmy began.

"Hey, don't worry. I don't need an answer right now. But the sooner the better," Colton said.

He was sure he had gotten his point across, judging by the worried look on Jimmy's face. Out of the corner of his eye, he saw Rubano heading toward him.

"Hey, Colton—"Rubano began.

"Rubano, I want you to meet a friend of mine, or should I say a friendly competitor of mine, Jimmy Kirk. Jimmy here owns Global Med Distributors. Jimmy, this is Rob Rubano, medical correspondent for NBC. I think you're just the kind of guy he wants to talk to," Colton said.

"Hey Jimmy. I'm looking for a background source, maybe technical reference on all of this. Mind if we talk?" said Rubano.

Jimmy looked befuddled. Colton snickered and excused himself, leaving Jimmy to deal with the annoying Rubano. He got back to his seat just in time for the afternoon round of speakers.

***

The specialists took over for the afternoon's summit session. From their presentations, Colton guessed that the FDA and CDC had been looking at the prescription drug supply for about two weeks now, enough time to do some lab work and maybe rack up a few preliminary investigations, but not nearly enough time to draw too many hard conclusions. Now he knew for certain that if he cleaned up his supply, they would never be on to him, especially since he always made sure that his paperwork was perfect. The FDA would waste their time trying to track the source of the adulteration to the manufacturers first and wouldn't even begin to look at distributors until they had completed the sample testing and proven that the product was clean when it left the manufacturers. By that time, everything in the warehouses and pipeline would be clean, one hundred percent pure legitimate and all he had to do was lay low until the FDA found someone to pin this on. Then, he could resume his regular program.

Senator Conroy resumed the podium after the specialists finished, so Colton headed out the door to retrieve his car. He had seen and heard enough for one day. Now he needed to double check on Jackie. He knew he had to be cautious for the next few months, but he was confident that the trail would lead a long way away from him. By his estimate, this whole thing would blow over in a couple of weeks. He'd be back to his old production levels in about six months.

Out on the street, Colton called Jackie.

"What's going on?"

"Everything's fine. I got legitimate domestic on its way to Jersey," said Jackie.

"Why Jersey? Just have it sent to Malvern," Colton questioned.

"Can't do that, trust me. I'm delivering to Jersey, and then I'll have it brought up to Malvern."

"Jackie—"

"Colton, trust me, we'll talk detail later. I know what I'm doing here."

Colton was tired of fighting with Jackie, tired from his whole day. Just this once he would trust him and get the details tomorrow.

"We'll talk tomorrow. I need you to do me a favor. Call Betsy and tell her to find out about a Kat Vasquez, pharmacist in Maryland… first name might be Katherine, Kathleen, something with a 'K', I think—I don't know. Call me when you find something."

***

Kat returned to the summit and found a seat far from where she had been sitting. She wanted to avoid both Jimmy and Colton Barnes. She listened intently to the remainder of the speakers in the afternoon, taking copious notes and feeling her heart pound as she was again confronted with the scope of the problems in the drug supply.

The evidence seemed to point to a manufacturing issue or just plain counterfeits infiltrating the marketplace—only the lot testing and the records could prove that out. She was itching to get back to the hotel and go over the rest of the records she had from TemePhelps and either put them on the suspect list or move on to another manufacturer entirely.

She needed more information. While Senator Conroy grandstanded at the microphone, she made her way out of the room and down the hallway, pausing only briefly to hit the speed dial to Dan's direct line.

"How big do you know this thing to be?" she asked as Dan answered.

"I've got a feeling you're going to tell me now," he replied.

"I'm just leaving the Jefferson summit and we've got huge trouble, Dan. It's in every dosage form and pretty much in every class of drugs. It's much bigger than what international talked about," she said.

There was a long pause on Dan's end. Either he already knew the scope of the problem or he was caught off guard and didn't know what to say. She sincerely hoped that the latter was true.

"The field reports became more alarming over the past month," he finally said.

"National, or concentrated in one region?" she asked.

"Your region seems to be the hottest," he replied.

Kat let out a long sigh of exasperation. Maybe Dan had been reluctant to prejudice the investigators by letting out too much information, but Kat personally felt a bit ambushed now. Apparently she was heading up an inadequate team in the hottest spot in the country and she was let loose by HQ without any hint as to the scope of the problem. They were all going to pay for this blunder.

"I'm not sure how fast I can turn this around," she finally said.

"No one is. Listen Kat, it was too much to believe at once. We needed independent confirmation first. Now we have to fight for some more manpower. Sorry," he offered.

Kat stopped dead in her tracks. Her feelings of betrayal were tempered by the dread that now washed over her. She was in the middle of a crisis, the scope of which was ever growing and the boss had just so much as admitted that they were outgunned. She was trying to figure out just what to feel right now.

"Dan, how—" she began.

"Check with your team and see what they got today and let me know. We'll get on this," he cut in.

"Yep," she said quietly.

"Listen Kat, I want you to know we've got everyone working on this, as many bodies as we can possibly put on it," he offered.

"Let's just hope those bodies are faster than the ones that are dropping, huh?" she shot back.

Now Kat knew that the likely source of the crisis was in her region and that the problem was much more widespread than she first thought. She needed to forget about sleeping altogether and get as much done as she could in as little time as possible if she was going to get this stopped. As she walked to the truck, she could feel her knees weaken as the weight of the world settled in on her shoulders.

Once in the truck, she called Lonny and Tyrell and found out that they were on their way back from AmPharm and headed for the hotel. Kat called the front desk and rented another room in the hotel that they could use as a war room, someplace where the three of them could compare notes, brainstorm and hopefully quickly shut down whoever was poisoning America as fast as possible.

***

Colton checked his watch, hoping it was later than he thought it was. He really didn't want to get home in time for the wedding planner meeting, but it was only 3:30 and he was only a few blocks from the condo. He thought about heading over to Jersey to double check on Jackie's work, but decided to err on the side of caution. Everyone was on high alert and the last thing he needed was to be seen at a facility he didn't want anyone to know existed.

Cherie was in the kitchen fixing a pitcher of iced tea when he got there. He gave her a kiss and they briefly chatted about their day before he retreated to the bedroom to change. He heard the buzzer ring just as he was zipping up his jeans. He slipped on his loafers and headed for the front door. As he made his way down the hallway, Betsy called from the office. He quickly answered the call, and then asked her to hold for one minute.

"Colton, this is Jill Klinger from Platinum Events. Jill, my fiancé Colton Barnes," she said.

"Nice to meet you, Jill." Colton leaned in to shake her hand and took a good gaze at down her low-cut top. "I have to excuse myself and take an urgent call from the office," he said.

Colton headed into the office and shut the door before taking Betsy's call.

"Found an article on Vasquez's husband," Betsy said. "He was one of those people who got the diluted chemo a few years ago. Remember that? Anyway, I have a PDF I can send over if you want to read it."

"What's she doing now?" Colton asked.

"Still looking for that information," she replied.

"Call me when you get something," said Colton.

He hung up and waited to receive Betsy's email, although he didn't have to wait long. The article was from the Washington Post and detailed the court case that convicted pharmacist Joel Klein. He figured that was why Vasquez was interested in the Jefferson summit; she probably became some kind of crusader after the husband died. So, why was she in town the night of the Kammerly auction? He assumed Jimmy probably was sleeping with her and didn't want to talk about it.

"So where are we?" Colton asked as he joined Jill and Cherie in the living room.

"Venues. But I'm figuring on about three hundred and fifty guests—that sound right to you?" Cherie asked sweetly.

"Sounds about right," he replied, knowing that was the answer she wanted.

"Great! So, that narrows it down a little bit," said Jill.

He drifted off as the two women chatted what seemed like endlessly about the merits of one location over another. The more he mulled over the evidence, the more he was convinced that the Chinese were taking some of what was his supply and moving it directly to market under the manufacturer's name brand. He listed all the hard work, all the money it had taken him to create the perfect dies, the perfect formulations, and the perfect business plan. With each detail he grew angrier at whoever was damaging his perfect enterprise.

Chapter 8

Associated Press:

…According to researchers at Sloan Kettering, there has been a sharp increase in the fatality rate among cancer patients. Oncologists first believed they had encountered a more virulent form of the disease when fatality rates rose by about 25 percent. Concurrently, a sharp decline in chemotherapy effectiveness was noted. But, in spite of an increase in dosage rates and new and more potent drug cocktails, cancer fatality rates continued to rise. Researchers began testing the drugs themselves.

Nine out of ten samples of drugs revealed that only a fraction, anywhere from only 20 to 50 percent of the active ingredients, existed in the samples. Some of the drug was traced to smaller pharmacies specializing in chemotherapy that had deliberately diluted out the drug. In many of the additional cases, hospitals and cancer clinics discovered that the drugs from their supplies were adulterated. However, upon testing the suspect lots, results were found to be inconsistent as to the amount of active ingredient present, an indication that supplies may have originated from a number of different sources…

***

The night of the summit, Kat met with Lonny and Terrell to pull an all-nighter. But after hours of work, it was clear that their anger and adrenalin could not overcome just plain fatigue. Even the best brains needed to be cleared once in a while. The three broke ranks and planned to meet up in the morning.

Kat intended to sleep in, but landed in front of Albe's frat house first thing in the morning instead. She was never so happy to have slobber on her face. It seemed like a lifetime since she had last seen Bernie, even though it had only been a few days. The stress of the investigations and the recent revelations turned her into a mess that only a smelly, boisterous heap of a dog could fix.

"He's behaving?" she asked Albe.

"Yeah. But you must not be. No offense Mom, but you look like shit."

Kat chuckled and looked down at her wrinkled, ill-fitting slacks, baggy shirt, and scuffed shoes.

"Yeah. Tough few days," she mumbled. She could no longer resist Bernie's pull on the leash so she lurched forward to move along with him. Albe followed.

"So, am I allowed to ask?"

"What?"

"Whatever it is that has you looking like shit."

Kat wanted to answer, but knew that she could not. At least, not yet. The sun rose higher in the morning sky as Kat and Albe walked Bernie through the West Philadelphia neighborhood to a nearby park.

"You know I can't talk about it, Albe."

"I know. Just though it would help to ask. I heard about the summit. Scary stuff."

"That was not even the half of it."

"I don't understand how that happens. How does that happen? Are you guys asleep or something?"

Kat overlooked his righteousness; she was just too tired for an argument.

"The laws don't have any teeth and no one wants to pass one that does. And yet, they want the protection from a law that can't be enforced. Oh, and that's besides not having enough personnel."

"Sorry, Mom," he said without a hint of sarcasm.

Kat looked at Albe. He pretended to focus on the sidewalk ahead of them.

"Whatever. I should be glad that I'm stuck in town near you and Bernie, huh?"

The streets were full of traffic making their way to Center City for work, but somehow the atmosphere still seemed tranquil. Bernie bucked up and down on his hind legs, and then buried his face in the grass, ears flapping, hot on the scent of some vermin. Either the boys were not walking him or they didn't enforce proper leash behavior and Kat struggled to restrain the hound that was now twisting and jumping, bellowing up a tree. As annoying as Bernie was, for a few short minutes, Kat escaped the faces of the sick and dying that now haunted her.

She was surprised and impressed at the work that Tyrell and Lonny had done in her absence, and even more impressed at how they were able to work together and flesh out some pretty reliable leads. Today's plan was to split up and continue the investigations and if lucky, shut somebody down by the end of the week.

"Well Mom, I'm sure you'll be on to something soon," Albe suddenly said.

Kat smiled, and then found herself discussing the case with him, in spite of the little voice in her head chiding her for lack of professionalism. She must have needed to talk and whom more could you trust than your own son? They yanked Bernie down from the tree and kept walking toward a playground of brightly painted jungle gyms and swing sets.

"It's not accidental. Someone is deliberately and systematically moving counterfeits into the legitimate drug supply," she said.

"What about lot testing and tracking and all that?" Albe asked.

"They're forging it," she replied.

"Financials?" he asked.

Kat stepped back and took a look at her son, the one she thought never paid a bit of attention to what she did. He took the leash from her and tried to untangle Bernie, who had gotten himself wound around some playground equipment.

"They must have two sets of books. They're no irregularities in what we're seeing, so whoever this is knows the legitimate business from the inside. They're able to combine an illegal enterprise with the legitimate business and hide it very well," she said.

"So, they're probably someone already in the legitimate side of the business," Albe concluded.

"It would make the most sense," Kat replied.

"Yeah, but still, they've got to have a lot of extra money. Either they hide it or they're totally conspicuous, like Klein…"

As soon as the words left Albe's mouth, he stopped. It was the first time Kat could recall him even referring to his father's murderer and now the reference hung between them heavy and hard. They stood facing one another as Bernie bounced between them. Neither one noticed.

"I thought that if I became an FDA investigator, I would single handedly shut down all the Kleins of the world before they had a chance to hurt or kill anyone else," Kat said.

"It wasn't your fault, Mom. Dad knew that," said Albe.

Kat let the tears come for once.

"I still miss him. Maybe not as often or not as deeply, but I still miss him. I wonder sometimes what a day would feel like not missing him," she said.

"Me too."

Kat looked at her son, her only child from the love she shared with Jorge, and saw both the beginnings of a grown man and the lingering image of a child who was touched by a deep loss of a father long before any child should have been. Bernie walked toward her and Albe followed.

"You'll find them. You will Mom."

Bernie leaned up against her leg. His wagging tail slapped against the backs of her knees.

"Mmmm…"

"In the meantime, you're doing everything you can. I believe that," said Albe.

He put his arm around her and pulled her close to him for a moment, and then let go, but remained standing close enough to almost touch. Kat swelled with pride and silently mentioned to Jorge how proud he should be of his son. The two walked back to the frat house with Bernie in tow.

"You want to come by for dinner tonight? Martha's cooking," he asked.

"Absolutely," Kat replied.

She said a slobbery goodbye to Bernie and started to leave when Albe suddenly reached out and gave her another big hug. She held on tight as long as she could, but almost as fast as he had reached out to her, he stepped back and took off into the house without looking back.

Kat stood for a while, savoring the memory of him, imagining what it would have been like to stand there and watch him with Jorge at her side. For that moment, Jorge was very real to her again and his image rejuvenated her, rather than making her sad. She knew she had crossed some kind of line that separated her past from her present, her life from her hopes and dreams. It felt good.

She felt ready to meet back up with Tyrell and Lonny at the hotel and finalize the day's revisit of NorthAmerican-Genberg, check on a few more leads, and hopefully get some test results back from HQ. She was preoccupied with her thoughts as she got on the elevator at the hotel and hardly noticed when Jimmy Kirk stepped inside with a crowd of other people. It wasn't until she was almost at her floor, and the elevator had emptied out that she looked up and noticed him standing next to her.

"Got time for breakfast?" he asked as the elevator doors opened.

Kat stepped out and he followed close behind. She waited for the elevator doors to close before speaking.

"Jimmy, I—"

"It's just breakfast, Kat. Promise," he said.

"I'm a mess, I gotta get changed, and then I have meetings—"

"I'll wait in the lobby if you want," he offered.

He leaned close to her. She could smell his cologne and feel his desire for her. She tried her best to resist. When the time was eventually right, she knew they would be good together, but now she needed to concentrate on her work. Yet, her mind wandered back to their first night together and how much she had missed intimacy since Jorge's death. Now, she hesitated at the door, deciding whether to slide her card and unlock the lock or send him away before then. His hand landed on hers and then she knew the answer.

Kat was in the shower afterwards, energized for the rest of the day. For the first time in her life, she didn't second-guess her decision, but took it for what it was: a satisfying interlude that she richly deserved. Now she had work to do and ran down the list of what needed to be covered at her meeting with Lonny and Tyrell. She donned the hotel bathrobe and headed for the desk in the room for her phone.

"Your phone's been buzzing away the whole time you were in the shower. Must be urgent," said Jimmy. He headed into the bathroom and she checked her voice mails.

There three messages from Dan. Things were heating up in Washington. She put down the phone and quickly dressed; she just couldn't envision herself having a serious conversation with Dan wearing nothing but a bathrobe.

Dan picked up on the second ring. "Kneeley's on the warpath and firing up the whole Congressional committee. Boss man Eiser has issued an order for me to head up there with him and meet with him. Kat, I need to throw them a bone. You got anything I could let out now?"

"Nothing solid yet. I've got some good leads and a few hunches, but so far, nothing consistent has shown up in the testing or the inspections. We're pretty sure we've eliminated the manufacturers. Now we're looking at the distributors. But you know it's a huge job."

"I need you to go up there with me Kat. These guys are looking for blood and I need to produce some detail and somebody from the field to calm them down."

Kat wanted to scream. She couldn't imagine how she was going to fit one more thing into her day or what she had to lose sight of in order to turn in a command performance for the Congressional Committee head.

"What time's the meeting?" she asked.

"One o'clock," he replied.

Kat looked at her watch. The drive to D.C. would take her at least three hours and it was nine o'clock now. She had to hustle. She suddenly felt embarrassed that she had spent the morning on her own private pleasure instead of doing her job. Now she had to think fast and work faster.

"I'll be there," she said.

"Just don't come empty handed," he replied.

She was rushing around the hotel room, changing into her best black suit and getting organized enough to be able to talk to Lonny and Tyrell in the car, when Jimmy spoke.

"Things are heating up, huh?"

Kat jumped. She had completely forgotten that Jimmy was there.

"Congressional Committee," she mumbled.

"So, you guys are looking at distributors, huh?" he asked.

As soon as he asked the question, Kat stopped and closed her eyes, acutely aware of what she had just done.

"I gotta go, Jimmy," she said.

She had to get out of there before she said another word that Jimmy Kirk should not have heard. She finished dressing, packed up her notes and started to leave, and then suddenly stopped. Not only should she not have let Jimmy into the room, but also she certainly couldn't leave him in there now. She motioned him to the door.

"Hey, yeah, I gotta go. Got an appointment today that I can't be late for. See you tonight?" he asked.

"I don't know about tonight. Dan's on the hot seat and I gotta get down to D.C. and face the committee with him today," she said.

"Call me?" he asked.

Kat nodded.

"Will you?" he asked again.

"Sure," Kat said, unable to look him in the face.

She finally looked up to see Jimmy staring at her with one raised eyebrow. They both knew they couldn't see each until after the investigation was over, maybe not ever again. She wanted to give over to him, but the timing was lousy and the reality of their positions was worse. Maybe she was a little grateful for the excuse.

She smiled and he smiled back. He kissed her; she kissed him back halfheartedly. Then he left. It felt good to have Jimmy around, felt even better that he so wanted to have her around, but she knew now that it was over. She had to shove unprofessional thoughts of Jimmy Kirk into the dark recesses of her head.

Once in the car, she called Albe.

"I'm sorry, but I'm not going to make it to dinner tonight. I gotta head back to D.C. today for a meeting. I'll be back later, but things are kind of popping now. Tell Martha I'm sorry," she said.

"Mom, hang on," he said.

Kat listened and heard Albe jostling the phone around. Then, he finally spoke.

"Sorry, I was in class—"

"Shit Albe, don't leave class—"

"No, Mom, this is important. I was going to call you. I don't know why I didn't mention it before. Colton Barnes. You know that name?"

"I've heard it." Kat was cautious.

"Guy's a bigger legend than his father around here. Major drug lord, for years, and all under coach Daddy's nose. People even say some of Daddy's football team bought off him. It was all over a few years before I even got here, but people still talk about him like he's a god. There are even some guys here now trying to rival his enterprise."

"Okay Albe, that's interesting and all—"

"There was a profile of him in *Philadelphia Magazine,* about him being part owner of one of the largest wholesale distributorships on the east coast. You don't think it's suspicious that a notorious street drug dealer goes into the legitimate drug business?"

Kat tensed up. It was tempting to follow Albe, but this could all be legend and gossip. She needed real answers, real leads and real proof.

"Albe—"

"I gotta get back to class. But, you know he's the guy, Mom. You know it," he said.

Kat chuckled a little. It was so much easier to be definite when you're young. Maybe Albe had a point, one that was already on her radar, but she'd already jeopardized the case once and she wasn't going to chance it again. She called Tyrell.

"I gotta head back to D.C. today, but I'll be back later," she said.

"Ohhh, Kneeley and the boys getting anxious?" Tyrell said in his best Louisiana drawl, which made Kat smile.

"Exactly. I need you and Lonny to check out a few things for me right now and call me in the car."

Kat was about to rattle off the list in her head when Tyrell interrupted.

"We're already on it," he said.

"On what?" she asked, slightly incredulous.

"The hijacking," he said.

Kat almost lost control of the truck. She grabbed the wheel hard and slowed enough to get full control.

"What?! Where?"

"Tractor-trailer with pharmaceutical delivery hijacked in New Jersey. Not sure who's it was or if it was a private hauler, but they forced him off the road, came up with their own tractor, and took his trailer full of deliveries," said Tyrell.

"Shit!" she said.

"Yeah, shit is right. I don't even want to think about what might be comin' next," Tyrell added.

Kat surely didn't want to think about what might be coming in her meeting once the Committee got wind of this.

"Tyrell, I need you and Lonny to work on something for me. Owner of USA Distributors is Barnes. First name is Colton. Check with your contacts and see what you can find out about the guy. Ask Lonny to look into USA Distributors' history, see if there's anything fishy going on there."

"You sound like you know somethin' more than you're tellin'," he said.

"Just a hunch," answered Kat.

She was beginning to believe that it was more than just a hunch, but she needed something concrete before she hit the Beltway. If Lonny and Tyrell could find out enough in the next two hours to satisfy the committee and keep things out of the press, they could make a move on the guy. It was tough. The press was hot on the story now. The headlines in all the papers and on all the news stations were ramping up the hysteria. When Kat had checked the FDA site this morning, the incident report numbers had jumped another few hundred. The statistics were tough enough to take, but all over the news were the wrenching first hand stories from victims— mothers, fathers, sons and daughters, each stunned, sobbing and bewildered that the medications they rely on were killing them. Kat berated herself again for spending time with Jimmy.

***

The flight to St. Bart's was turbulent, the weather in St. Bart's was unusually cold and rainy, and Colton was already in a foul mood. As much as he wanted to cancel the morning's trip, it was out of the question. He needed to meet the Chinese in a secluded place, somewhere away from the ever-present eyes of investigators, somewhere the Chinese could either confess to elbowing in on his market or point a finger at those who were.

The Chinese loved to talk about their business philosophy—"relationship building" they called it—and Colton learned early it meant they made money off your hide any way they wanted, including stealing. They were guarded about themselves and never revealed secrets, were hardly ever truthful even about their own names, and yet, they demanded to know every bit of your operation. Colton understood this. He knew the tricks and had spent time on their own turf. But Tsang and Ho were liaisons assigned to him by Mr. Chen in China and he knew little about them. He could have tried to strong arm Mr. Chen for answers, but he knew full well that Chen would tip off Tsang and Ho. Then, there was no telling what they would do. Instead, he would try to get them to tip their own hand, knowing the one thing the Chinese loved to do was brag.

He brought Reggie, Gus, and Stewart for protection and in case additional persuasion was needed. He was still considering which way to play his hand with them—cool and subtle or like a sledge hammer. The answer would come as the encounter progressed, and he had briefed Reggie and the others to be ready either way.

Though his mind was firmly focused on his meeting, just being in St. Bart's was distracting, relaxing, making it hard to focus on his mission. He was anxious to see his gardens again, maybe even get a chance to work in them if the dreary weather dissipated. He often found himself tense now—not just because of the pressure from business but also from the consequences of giving Cherie a ring. The wedding talk and planning was annoying but it was the change in Cherie, her new boldness that bothered him the most. There were moments he was about to put her back in her place, but he would catch himself and remember how much he needed her, especially now. He was feeling the pressure of losing control of his carefully designed business model, his carefully designed personal life, and his carefully designed life.

Reggie pulled up in the rental car, opened the door for Colton, tossed his bag in the trunk, and took off for the villa. His meeting was scheduled for an hour from now, with just enough time for him to try to relax and the guys to grab something to eat before they all met up at the business villa. They would get there on time; Tsang and Ho would be late. The Chinese were always late, deliberately late. They believed they controlled their opponent if they showed up on their own timetable. He could deal with the lateness, it was the assumption that he was too stupid to recognize what they were doing that enraged him. He devised his own way to win at their game: for every one minute they kept him waiting, he would keep them waiting for two. By his calculation, his meeting wouldn't get started for another two and a half hours. He would use the time to plan strategy with Reggie and the others.

The villa was in splendid order, as usual, and Colton nibbled at some food before settling into a chair and snapping on CNN. The lead story was some nonsense about the death of a young actress from an accidental overdose of drugs and alcohol, which made him laugh. Back in his high school and college dealing days, he'd supplied actors and actresses, athletes, politicians and wealthy brats, all of the same ilk as the dead girl on the television. He thought of all of them as pathetic, victims of their own stupidity, and suckers for using their leisure time to make him rich. He was about to turn the channel when the headline story switched to coverage of the Jefferson summit. Colton turned up the volume and sat forward in his chair.

The reporter was interviewing Dan Smithson, head of the investigations unit of the FDA and showing a montage of file photos of Smithson at congressional hearings or at press conferences. As he watched, Colton thought he spotted a familiar face in the background. He hit the speed dial for Betsy and hardly waited for her to answer before plunging in.

"Find out where to look up FDA investigators," he said.

"Right now?" she asked.

"Now!" he shouted.

Colton heard Betsy tapping on her computer keys, mumbling to herself.

"Okay. So, I found where I could look up an investigator on the FDA's website," she said.

She sighed heavily and Colton could hear the annoyance in her tone.

"Kat Vasquez," he said.

"Oh, we're back to her. Hang on." Betsy came back on the line quickly. "Okay… let's see…Lead investigator, Atlantic region, based out of FDA headquarters in Maryland."

Colton slammed his fist on the cushion. He knew he had a sixth sense about her, knew that his gut was always right. Now he wondered how long she'd been working the area.

"Get Jackie to call me *now!*" he yelled.

Colton tossed his phone on the couch, reached for the remote, and turned up the volume on the television. He was only partially relieved to see that the story focused on manufacturers. Counterfeits were only fleetingly mentioned. The FDA was targeting manufacturers and raw goods imported into the country, which meant he had to look out for his containers in port. His phone rang just as the piece ended.

"What's up?" Jackie asked, sounding too casual.

"FDA's going to be all over us soon," he said.

"Okay, we're ready," Jackie replied.

Jackie's blasé demeanor grated on Colton.

"What the fuck are you doing to make sure we're ready?!" he screamed.

"Calm down, Colton," said Jackie.

"Don't tell me to fucking calm down! How do you not get how serious this is? Huh? What, now you don't have any answers?" he screamed.

"You want to listen now? We're moving the rest of the mixed goods out of the pipeline and back to Jersey today and replacing with all new goods," Jackie said.

Colton paced the room to calm himself and took his time before answering.

"Unmarked trucks, right?" he finally said.

"Always," Jackie replied.

Jackie was just too confident, just too controlled. Colton snapped off the television, sighed heavily, and rubbed his eyes.

"This is no time to play, Jackie," he growled.

"I swear Colton, it's under control. Nothing to worry about," Jackie said.

A silence hung between them as Colton calculated how fast he could get back to Philadelphia after his meeting.

"How's the meeting going?" Jackie asked, breaking the silence.

"Hasn't happened yet. Jackie, the FDA's crawling through the area now. It may have been here for at least a week already. They're coming in one day soon, any day."

"Colton, I'm telling you it's not going to be a problem."

"Your life's on that," said Colton.

Jackie didn't answer.

"You hear what I said?!" he screamed.

"Got it," Jackie finally said.

Colton hung up, then pounded down a couple of stiff drinks trying to calm himself. He drained his glass and threw it into the wall. Pieces of glass flew around the room. The front door opened and Reggie peeked his head in.

"I need you guys in here!" Colton screamed.

Reggie and the others sauntered into the living room of the villa and took up seats on the couch and the side chairs. They seemed serious, but Colton was so agitated now that if any of them did the slightest thing to annoy him, he was going to pop them in the face with his fist. They were perfectly behaved—like schoolchildren in front of the principal, quietly waiting for him to speak.

"No matter which way these fucks come at us, we will have the upper hand. Got it?" he said.

A rumble of "okay," "sure" and "yes, boss" came back.

"That includes making one of them disappear," he said.

This time the crew held perfectly still, hardly breathing. Only Reggie faintly nodded in response.

Colton bore his eyes into each one of them until he was sure they understood his message. As he did, each one offered a nod, a faint smile or some kind of gesture of confirmation. Once he was satisfied he had made his point, he moved on to strategy.

Colton and Reggie plotted for the next hour, covering every last detail of the meeting with the Chinese. Two and a half hours later, long after the scheduled meeting time, they all made their way up the road to the business villa. Tsang and Ho were not there. Colton took up his usual chair on the far side of the room to wait. Reggie took up one side of the room, Gus on the other. Stewart positioned himself near the door.

About fifteen minutes later, Tsang and Ho arrived. Reggie allowed them into the room, patted the two down and confiscated their weapons, and then ushered the two men back outside and stayed with them. Gus surveyed the weapons and told Colton that they had come with serious firepower, so Colton gave the signal to handle the two with force. Gus and Stewart nodded and radioed the plan to

Reggie's earpiece. Another agonizingly long thirty minutes passed before Colton gave the signal to allow the two men in. The door opened and Tsang and Ho stepped inside, followed closely by Reggie.

There was only one chair in the room, the one in which Colton sat, so Tsang and Ho were forced to stand. They stood defiantly, chins up, legs wide, and shoulders square.

"Gentlemen, I don't have time to waste, so we'll settle this quickly. Get out of my business. Now," he said.

"We no sure what you talk about," said Tsang.

"Yes you are. You guys got greedy and decided to go out on your own. Into *my* fucking markets!" he shouted.

"You have wrong information," said Ho, jutting his chin out even further.

"No. I don't. Your stuff is junk. I don't peddle junk and I don't dump junk. I work a clean operation. Now I've got a lot of unpleasant attention focused on me because of you," Colton spat.

"Maybe your competitors are to blame," said Ho.

Colton planted himself in his chair, knowing that he had to resist his overwhelming urge to lunge forward and strangle the man with his bare hands.

"I. Would. Know. If. That. Were. True," he growled.

"We have heard many things. Maybe more things than you have heard," said Ho, relaxing his stance into a slump.

Colton clenched his teeth and balled and unballed his fists.

"How much crap are you guys moving directly into my markets?" he demanded.

"We still don't—"

Colton burst out of his seat and charged at Ho. Reggie, Gus and Stewart rushed forward to back him up, but Colton stopped himself before he assaulted the man; instead, he stood close, his face inches from Ho's and hissed his words through his teeth. Ho never flinched.

"How much? I know you're masquerading as manufacturers, dumping your junk on guys who don't know better, the same junk that isn't good enough to make into my operation. The only way you're even getting anything at all is out of *my* plants in China. I bought and paid for those plants. They're mine! So whatever little friends you made with my guys in China is over. Now. Got it?" he said.

"Our operation—"

"STAY THE FUCK OUT OF MY BUSINESS!" Colton suddenly screamed.

Reggie, Gus and Stewart stepped even closer. Colton shoved Tsang back, then slugged Ho in the gut. He stepped back and let Gus and Steward grab the guys and hold them still.

"We are not sure what—" Ho began.

"Your junk brought investigators right to our doorstep! Understand? Comprendo? Huh? I DON'T GIVE A FUCK ABOUT YOU OR YOUR OPERATION. I WANT YOU OUT OF MINE!" he screamed.

Colton stood close to Tsang and Ho, breathing hard, feeling the blood course through his veins. He now he had to make a bold statement or these guys would only be the beginning of many more to come. Taking them both out was too risky, but killing one would send a clear message back to China. Colton raised his hand and pointed to Ho, and then took one step to the side and headed for the door. Behind him, he could hear a scuffle and the two men at first speaking, then yelling to one another in Chinese. Finally, he heard Ho's voice yelling at him in English.

"We are many and you are so few," Ho said, laughing.

Colton called out over his shoulder without even looking back at Ho, "You're just another dead man." On his way out the door, he heard the distinct crunch of breaking bones. Colton knew Tsang would watch Ho die.

***

Kat met Dan outside Kneeley's office in Senate Russell Office Building a half hour before the scheduled meeting. Dr. Eiser, Commissioner of the FDA and Dan's boss, was already inside with the Senator. It was clear that the Senator's aides were restricting Dan from entering the office until the Commissioner and the Senator deemed it necessary and they weren't being very congenial about it. The stress was clearly wearing on Dan. His face was drawn, his color pallid. Kat so wished that she could have marched down the hallway and met him with the news that the culprit was caught and within days the drug supply would be secured and returned to safety. Unfortunately, though Tyrell and Lonny were able to make some progress, without a thorough inspection of USA Distributors and interrogation of Barnes, most of what Kat was able to bring to Dan were only leads— good, hard leads, but just leads.

"So, how confident are you that this is the guy?" Dan asked.

"Eighty percent. Tyrell called in some street sources and got some pretty hard stuff on this guy, Barnes," she said.

Dan massaged the bridge of his nose and sighed.

"Is it going to stick?" he asked.

"Always the question, Boss," said Kat.

"What about the partner? Can you make a deal with him?" Dan asked.

"Haven't gotten to him yet. We're scheduled to get in there as soon as I can get back. Can't speculate on how much cooperation we can get out of him, but we'll try our best," she said.

Dan nodded. He paced a few steps across the hall and back again.

"Where's the supply coming from?" he asked.

"Pretty sure it's Chinese. High quality counterfeits, impressive really. Somebody got inside and reproduced the dies exactly, matched colors, pretty dead on. Problem is, there's also some evidence that there are multiple sources.

Once we get into the distribution site, we'll be able to tell," she answered.

"You're convinced it's not a manufacturer?" he probed.

"Pretty well convinced. Distributor would explain the longer time frame, the spotty and varied interactions, maybe even some of the lot testing results," she answered.

Kat could tell that Dan was close to his breaking point and she hoped that he would catch a second wind before they had to face Senator Kneeley. Much as she was glad to be here to help Dan out, she wanted to be back with Lonny and Tyrell working the case and making sure she could shut down Colton Barnes.

"Sorry it's taking so long, Dan."

"Hey, I know how thorough you are. More important to get it right than grab the headline."

Kat could tell that something else was bothering Dan. He had never been concerned about facing the Senator or the Committee, he was always the outspoken guy on the Hill. Today he just looked tired and sad.

"Everything all right?" she asked.

He hesitated at first, then quietly spoke.

"I lost my dad day before yesterday," he answered.

"Oh, Dan. I'm so sorry—"

Dan held up his hand and shook his head. Kat fell silent.

"He'd had some heart issues, but he threw a clot. I know it was the bad Coumadin, Kat. Can't let that slip to my mom, it would kill her. But I know it was," he said.

Kat resisted the temptation to reach out and hug him.

Dan stepped closer to her, took a deep breath and paused. He finally spoke.

"We gotta get it stopped, Kat."

Suddenly Kat felt the full weight of everything crashing down on her. Even the Investigative Director of the FDA had lost his father. It's a sacred trust the distributors are charged with and yet they were the weakest link in the entire chain, and no one, in spite of their continuing rhetoric, had the courage to take them on. No matter how indignant the Senators and the committees and even the President want to get, until they translated their indignation into legislation that will really protect the American people, it all amounted to just more rhetoric. Kat wasn't sure how much of what she was thinking would come out of her mouth at the meeting and she cautioned herself to swallow those words.

"The Senator's ready to see you now," announced one of the aides.

Kat followed Dan into the office, biting the sides of her tongue almost hard enough to make them bleed.

The snotty aide ushered them through the waiting area and into Senator Kneeley's office. Kneeley sat in a high backed leather chair behind the huge, wooden desk, absorbed in whatever he was reading, with his glasses perched on the end of his nose, and a plastic Bic pen in his hand. He was as much of a rumpled mess as his office. Floor to ceiling bookshelves were jammed full and every flat surface of the room was covered with stacks of papers. Commissioner Eiser sat in one of the four chairs in front of the desk and the other chairs were filled by men in suits. A gaggle of aides clustered in the back corner of the office. One of the aides motioned for Dan and Kat to take up seats on the paper and notebook-covered couch against the wall. The two squeezed onto the couch between the obstacles while the aides watched and snickered.

"Commissioner, please tell Senator Kneeley what progress has been made in this investigation," said one of the aides as though the Senator wasn't even in the room and able to speak for himself.

The Commissioner began to address Senator Kneeley, unphased by the fact that the question came from an aide at the back of the room. "Well, the reports I'm receiving from Investigative Director Smithson—"

"You Smithson?" Kneeley asked, pointing his Bic at Dan.

"Yes, Senator," Dan answered.

"Good, fine. We don't have to be so formal here. Just tell me, what's the latest news on this thing?" asked Kneeley.

Dan relaxed his shoulders. "We've got all the agents in the field that we can spare, most of them concentrated in the Mid-Atlantic region where we think the problem is originating," Dan answered.

"This thing is, is getting worse?" asked Kneeley.

"We've had more cases in the last few days—"

"To be exact: another five hundred reported cases of interactions and about twenty-five more deaths just in the last three days," interjected one of the snot-nosed aides.

Kat narrowed her eyes at the aide.

"Ah, that right?" the Senator asked.

"Yes, Senator," Dan answered.

Kneeley raised his eyebrows and peered first at Eisen, and then at Dan.

"Senator, Dan and his investigative unit—" began Commissioner Eisner.

"You in the field?" Kneeley asked Kat, ignoring the Commissioner.

She felt her heart jump when he addressed her directly.

"Philadelphia," she answered.

"And, what is the latest, ah, latest information?" he asked.

"We've got a solid lead on a distributor we think is responsible. My agents are working contacts as we speak and we're poised to conduct an on-site today, as soon as I get back," she replied.

"How, ah, solid do you think this lead is?" he probed.

"We're pretty confident—"

One of the men in suits began barking immediately, "Don't you think the time for *pretty* confident has passed? After all, you guys have known about this for months. Ed, we're not going to sit here and be the victims of some witch-hunt that makes our manufacturers and distributors look bad. You can't pin this thing on us just because the FDA can't manage to do its job right."

Kat glanced at Dan, who seemed confused, and then to Eisen, who was either resigned or bored. Couldn't they see this was an ambush? Kat found herself talking back to the guy before she could stop.

"With all due respect, sir, I wonder whether any of you here have ever conducted an investigation with few tools and even fewer resources. Investigators go out there with the knowledge that our back-breaking efforts to expose the criminal entity can't be enforced because guys like you get paid to come in here and convince Congress that any kind of legislation is a burden on your industry!"

Dan tapped Kat's foot with his. She knew as soon as the words flew out of her mouth that she needed to stop, but once she started, she wasn't going to back down.

"Miss whatever your name is, the pharmaceutical industry is already choking on regulation. The fact that some rogue criminal tainted the supply doesn't mean that the government needs carte blanche in plastering more regulation that will endanger the health of the American people," yapped another suit.

"Does anyone remember the Tylenol disaster?" asked a third. "Cost the industry millions in lost revenue, not to mention what it now has to spend on tamper-proof packaging, for no good reason. Just some crazy out there with a grudge."

Kat didn't even try to control herself anymore.

"You guys have done everything you could to protect your profits and *only* your profits, not to mention your CEO bonuses. The last thing you care about is protecting the American public or developing drugs to help the American people!"

Kat hoped she hadn't gotten anyone fired, including herself. She forced herself to stay in her seat when everything in her wanted to march across the room and thump those guys in the head. She gulped a few deep breaths and forced herself to look at Kneeley and see how much damage she had done. Unbelievably, he didn't register any kind of annoyance, unlike Eiser, whose neck was crimson.

Dan glanced at Eiser, and then leaned forward to addressed Kneeley directly, "Kat Vasquez is one of our very best investigators who takes her job very seriously—"

"Senator," she interrupted, "I'm not going to let Dan take the fall for me. I apologize for my lack of diplomacy. But, as a pharmacist, I swore an oath and I take that Pharmacy Oath very seriously. Every one of those names of the dead and the injured are seared into my memory just as if they were my own family. Baby Emma, Mr. Wilbert, Jack and Sarah and little Shayna from 16th Street Elementary--"

The Senator put up his hand to stop Kat. The room was still silent.

"I won't stop until I get whoever's doing this. The only way to insure there won't be another criminal taking over as soon as we stop this one is to finally get serious about some legislation. I'm not telling you anything you don't already know."

A cacophony of voices rose up after that. Kat braced herself for what was to come next. Kneeley seemed content to allow the arguing to continue, while he impassively peered over his glasses at each speaker.

Finally, Kneeley's voice rose above the din. "I've heard enough. We need to let this investigator get on with her work. You'll have something concrete in the next day or so, correct Miss Vasquez?"

"Hopefully sooner," Kat replied, grateful that the Senator did not take the opportunity to grandstand nor to chide her and the department.

"Let's find out who's doing this first, and then decide how to prevent it from happening again," said Kneeley. He motioned to the aides in the back of the room and they sprang into action opening the door and ushering everyone out. The Lobbyists left first, followed by

Commissioner Eisner; Dan and Kat brought up the rear. Before they got out of the room, Kneeley spoke again.

"Ah, Miss Vasquez," he began.

Kat braced herself and turned to face him. She hoped that at least she could finish out this case before she was banished from the department.

"Perhaps when this is all settled you can speak freely to the committee as we draft new legislation?" he asked.

Kat was stunned. She could only muster a silly grin as a response. She turned and followed the others out of the office and into the hallway. The Commissioner had already taken off to return to his office, but Dan had waited for Kat.

"Sorry Dan. I just couldn't sit back—"

"Don't apologize to me. It needed to be said. I reassigned all forces in the region to your command. They should be there when you get back. Good luck," he said.

Kat was proud that she had stood up and said what needed to be said and grateful that it didn't seem to put Dan in a tough spot. She continued to seethe about the lobbyists but then redirected her anger to Colton Barnes. She spent the drive time back running the details in her head, plotting a strategy of how to take on Barnes and USA Distributors and make sure that they were taken down correctly. Every time she thought of what all could go wrong, she remembered Dan's strained face, which began a parade of all the dead and injured that she couldn't shake from her mind. Those images drove her; was going to get restitution for every single one of them.

Lonny and Tryell were in the war room as soon as she got in.

"So, you guys got anything new for me?" she asked.

"Looks like Mr. Barnes spent some time in China and picked up a few business connections. Looks legit on the surface, but we're still digging," said Lonny.

"Plenty of verification on the street," chimed in Tyrell. "This guy's reputation precedes him. Charming and as mean as a snake in the garden of Eden. Hey, how'd the meeting go?"

"Well, I didn't get fired. Found out that Dan's father got caught in the Coumadin thing though. Died a couple of days ago," she said.

Lonny sighed loudly. Tyrell shook his head and whistled softly.

"So, what've we got?" she asked.

"Got more dead hens than we can count and only partial fox tracks," said Lonny.

"Now, what the hell does that mean?" asked Tyrell.

"Means the tracks could be a fox or they could be the family dog," replied Lonny.

Tyrell made a face and shook his head. Kat snickered at the two of them, a real odd couple, and sat down across from Lonny.

"I just need some facts, guys. We need to strike USA Distributors tonight but I need something hard to bring in local cops. They're not coming in on speculation and we can't get a warrant on a gut feeling," said Kat.

"Word on the street is that it's got all the branding of Barnes. But he may not be working alone," said Tyrell.

"Got hold of some security video from the parking lot camera at USA Distributors," Lonny said as he turned the laptop screen toward Kat. "Early morning meeting with this guy, Ji—"

"Jimmy Kirk." The words fell out of Kat's mouth before she could stop them.

"Pretty sure, yeah. One of the owners of GlobalMed, a distributor himself," said Tyrell.

Kat struggled to focus, to stifle the urge to bolt from the room.

"Now, this may mean something, or it may not…" said Lonny.

She tried to silence her thumping heart, afraid that Lonny and Tyrell could hear it from across the table. She bit the inside of her lip to prevent any more words from escaping from her mouth. She knew from the beginning that the encounter with Jimmy was foolish, but she didn't stop herself, and now she just handed the defense a reasonable doubt that could destroy the entire case. Lonny and Tyrell continued to speak, but the voice in her head was louder. Finally, she bolted out of her chair.

"Ah, listen," she blurted. "Let me take a minute, okay? It's been kind of a long day. I, ah, I just need a couple of minutes."

She barely made it to the bathroom in the hotel lobby before she doubled over in dry heaves and struggled to lock herself into a stall. Too many memories flooded back, too much guilt over naïve and lousy choices, first with Jorge and now with Jimmy. Now there were thousands of Jorges and another Kat Vasquez bad decision. She punched the side of the stall because she couldn't punch herself. It took some minutes for her to calm down enough to face herself in the mirror. But she could only glance at her reflection, utter a simple apology to the air and wash any expression off of her face. There was no time for self-pity; the time was needed to make sure Colton Barnes got shut down. Today.

A couple more OCI investigators were waiting in the USA Distributors parking lot when Kat and the others pulled in. Ten more regular investigators whom Dan had reassigned to the case arrived just after Kat parked the truck.

Tyrell gave her the particulars on Colton Barnes on the ride over. Turns out he was a rather infamous guy and many of the contacts, if not all, still revered his name and had plenty to tell. She had to marvel at the corruption within Philadelphia and suburban police departments that seemed to also know that the son of a big time football coach was dealing drugs right under their noses *for almost a decade* and no one every arrested him. Kat tried to control her incredulousness.

"If his skin was the color of mine they'd beat his ass and throw him in jail faster than your mama hit you with a switch," added Tyrell.

Kat was trying to stay professional, to keep herself from torching USA Distributors and hoping that Colton Barnes was locked inside. She was trying not to think of Jorge dying and Klein enjoying his lavish life or Colton

Barnes bragging about his cleverness. She was trying not to berate herself for Jimmy Kirk. Every time she was tempted to fly off halfcocked, she made herself remember that congressional committees and law enforcement prefer hard evidence to gossip.

They all assembled in the parking lot, with Kat briefing the other agents and everyone mapping out a strategy for working the facility.

"We have to move fast. If this dude gets one hint that we're on to him, he's got everything underground fast as you can blink," insisted Tyrell.

"The kid's right. We have to get there first, before we alert the police boys and before this guy calls in his buddies to hide him," added Lonny.

"How many men over at GlobalMed?" she asked.

"Half a dozen. They're positive Kirk's in the building and should be able to take him in easily," said Lonny.

Kat nodded. She pretended to check over her notes one last time but kept her head down until she had fully composed herself. She tried not to imagine how Jimmy was going to feel when a slew of cops showed up with handcuffs. Then she snapped to attention.

"Questions?" she asked, and then looked at each and every agent surrounding her. Each one nodded in return. Kat led the way to the front door.

***

The sun came out for the latter part of the day in St. Bart's and drove Colton out into the garden. The caretaker arrived as he was puttering. He was a young man with a cheerful smile and dark brown skin from his work in the sun.

"The plants are lovely this time of year," Colton said.

The man smiled and nodded appreciatively. Colton introduced himself and shook the man's hand, whose name he thought he heard to be Benoit.

"Merci, Mister Barnes," he said.

"I'm curious about the orchids. The rare ones thrive here, yes?" Colton asked. "Yes, yes, very much so," Benoit said, nodding.

He carefully cradled a cluster of flowers in his hands. Colton watched as he lovingly pinched off the spent flowers and removed any yellowed leaves from the plants.

"Government forbids me from having them at home," said Colton.

"I send to you," said Benoit.

Colton looked at Benoit and squinted. The man had read his mind.

"We cut out…eh, the grow parts…clumps, eh, clumps of orchid cells. Place on the agar. Wrap for you, no one looks. No one knows. This I do very well," he said.

Benoit smiled broadly at Colton and stood proud, acting out again how he would carefully remove the orchid plants from their host and properly package them for delivery.

"You could bring them to me yourself, huh?" asked Colton.

He figured it was better for Benoit to get caught smuggling rare orchids than himself.

"Yes, yes!" Benoit enthusiastically nodded.

"Good. I'll fly you to Philadelphia and you'll bring me orchids. You can see the ones I have in my collection," said Colton.

Now Benoit smiled and nodded so furiously that Colton thought his head would bob off. He shook the gardener's hand and told him they would work out the details before he left. The exchange put Colton in a better mood; so much better that he thought he might go down to the beach and retrieve one of the topless beauties for an afternoon screw.

He went back inside the villa and changed into his beach clothes, excited already at the prospect of a spending the rest of the day with a tanned beauty. He met Reggie at the car, climbed into the back, and told him to steer for

Grand Cul de Sac beach, where native girls and tourist beauties gravitated on the lookout for wealthy men.

"So, everything taken care of?" Colton asked Reggie as he pulled the car up to the front doors of Le Guanahani Hotel.

"Vanished without a trace," said Reggie.

"And the other one?" Colton asked.

"Loaded on a plane back to Philly."

"Good."

"You need me to wait here?" Reggie asked.

Colton shook his head. "I'll be awhile. Go back to the villa. I may call you later."

Colton checked in at the front desk and although he had no luggage, the bellman still escorted him up to the room and pointed out the particulars of the amenities. After pouring himself a drink from the bar and surveying the beach from his balcony for prospects, he headed downstairs.

He skipped the young women by the pool; they were usually there with a man or in a group. He had become lazy since Cherie and his skilled madams and wondered whether he had lost his touch altogether. He made his way down to the beach, scanning the pickings as he went, and then found an empty chaise next to one with the remnants of what were clearly a woman's things. Judging by the designer name on the beach bag and the sandals, this woman was young. He hoped she was also beautiful.

He waited for about ten minutes, pretending to be asleep while he squinted from behind his sunglasses at every woman who approached. Soon, the owner of the items showed up. She was perhaps in her late twenties, plain, but passable, without any inconvenient rings on her fingers. She wore a yellow and red patterned bikini, which only looked good on her from the waist up and she glistened with droplets of water from her dip in the ocean. Colton waited for her to settle back into her chaise before pretending to awaken from his nap.

"You speak English?" he asked.

She nodded.

"Thank goodness. I've been trying to find someone to talk to for the last couple of hours. Are you here with your family?" he asked.

She hesitated, and then finally replied.

"No."

Now he knew she was his. He sized her up as he continued to speak, gauging how much time it would take to get her into bed. She was not very beautiful—homely at some angles, with thighs that were too big for her small breasts. She would probably be quite willing to screw him once he began flashing around money. He ordered drinks from the hotel waiter and engaged her in small talk, concentrating on saying whatever would get her upstairs as quickly as possible. After another half hour, he made his move. He announced that he was going back to his room for a Jacuzzi and vaguely offered what she might have considered an invitation to join him. She showed little interest in his invitation, but he knew it was an act; as soon as he left, she would follow. He knew women needed to believe their encounters were somehow their idea. He had not even made it to the front door of the hotel before she had fallen in lockstep with him.

They rode the elevator exchanging silly conversation and he pretended that he was embarrassed at their soon-to-be encounter. As they entered his suite, he realized that he had forgotten to take his little blue pill, had even forgotten to bring them with him to the hotel. A slight feeling of panic rose up in him. He'd never had trouble with a stranger before and he made himself assume that he would not have trouble now.

She was impressed with the suite and became more flirtatious with the discovery of each additional room, each balcony, and each spectacular view of the beach below. Soon she had stripped down to just her bikini, standing close to him at the bar as he fixed her a silly island drink. He wished she had left her skirt on to cover her heavy thighs. He tried to focus only on her breasts.

He downed a shot of Scotch while she was in the bathroom, and then fixed himself a proper Scotch and soda on the rocks and stood looking as respectable as his drink. When she re-emerged from the bathroom, she retrieved her drink and hovered around him, sipping and circling, hesitating and then drawing even closer to him with each successive pass. For his part, he stood still and pretended to be patient, all the while feeling the familiar bulge between his legs, fantasizing about how wet she would be and how those too fleshy thighs would feel. Finally, she finished her drink, leaned over and planted a kiss on his mouth. She tasted like fruit punch and he wished that she tasted of something smokier, more sophisticated.

He led her into the bedroom where he sat her on the bed, and then leaned into her and gave her a slobbery kiss. She did just as he had hoped, undid his pants and took him in her mouth. She was pretty good with her mouth—good enough for him to forget his worries about his little blue pill. Once he was sure he was ready to perform, he laid her down on the bed and undid the bottom tie of her bikini top, slowly inching it up so he could see the red and yellow fabric tangled up around her neck. It was not as good as the necklace from the Palestinian, but it would work.

He removed her bikini bottoms, stripped himself naked, then climbed up on the bed to enter her. She reached up to pull his face down to kiss him. His instinct was to resist her, but he feared he would not get his way if he did not comply. After he entered her and their movements became faster, she reached up to remove the bikini top from her neck and he grabbed her hand hard, harder than he meant to. He saw the fear in her eyes. He loosened his touch until the fear left, and then felt obliged to kiss her again.

When it was over, he rolled off of her and wished for her to disappear. He was agitated now—satisfied but annoyed at the amount of work it took to get a girl here to screw and now how much it would take to get rid of her. These kinds of girls wanted to hang around, thinking they had a meaningful encounter and continuing to dream about the rich guy they met on vacation. This was why he almost always relied on professionals. Today he risked at regular girl and now he regretted it. He got up from the bed and walked to the shower where he scrubbed off her fruity smell and replaced it with the musky smelling hotel spa products. He exited the shower and wrapped himself in the hotel's luxurious terry robe, tying the belt tight around his expanding waist, and went back into the bedroom.

She was fast asleep on the bed with her mouth open in an unappealing way, snoring. It made him cringe to look at her. He scooped up his clothing from the floor and went into the living room where he quickly dressed, left the suite and checked out downstairs.

Back at the villa, he ordered food for himself and Reggie and sat back to relax. He reclined near the pool and watched the sun set across the ocean, remembering the vision of Cherie in this very spot, remembering how she was not long ago, wishing he could bring that old Cherie back. He felt the weight of too many annoyances these days—the Chinese, the FDA, the new Cherie. He started to think seriously about handing the business to Jackie. Maybe he would buy a mansion in the country and build greenhouses, like the DuPonts, and grow orchids and other rare flowers that would suit his fancy. His phone jarred him out of his fantasy. He checked the number before answering.

"This better be good, Jackie," he said.

"FDA just walked in," was the reply.

Colton sat bolt upright on the chaise and paced across the patio to the edge of the railing.

"How many?" he asked.

"Two guys," Jackie replied.

Colton relaxed. Two guys meant a routine inspection.

"Colton, I got this under control, remember? We're fine. I'll call you when I can. Just didn't want you to be surprised."

He hung up before Colton could reply. He paced the length of the deck, calculating how much time it would take to charter a jet back to Philadelphia.

"Reggie!" he screamed.

He appeared at the doors to the pool.

"We fly home tonight. Let the guys know."

He called Betsy and had her book a commercial flight back to Philadelphia for the four of them. Even if the FDA worked through the night, they would still need to be back at his facility tomorrow. He wanted to make sure he was there for at least some of the inspection. There was no way they could gain access to his books and his real supply chain, but he needed to size these FDA guys up.

***

Jackie DeAngelo met Kat and her team as soon as they entered. "Good evening," he said as he ushered them inside. "I'm Jackie DeAngelo, part-owner."

The guy was calm, relaxed. Almost cheerful. His clothes were too neat and pressed, no hint of five o'clock shadow—odd for a guy who'd been at work all day. The look of him didn't sit right with Kat.

"Here's the official inspection notification," she announced as she handed him paperwork.

"Thanks," Jackie said. He didn't even glance at the paperwork.

"You can look that over," Kat said, pointing.

"Oh, I'm sure everything's perfect. Just let me know what you need from me," he replied.

"It's all on the inspection notice," she said.

Finally, DeAngelo read over the paperwork, and then got on the phone and called in the appropriate representatives. Employees appeared within minutes of his call.

Lonny and Tyrell matched groups of agents with each of the employees and the groups dispersed throughout the facility. Only Kat remained with DeAngelo.

"Should the facility be placed on some kind of lockdown?" he asked.

She was curious about his suggestion and use of the word lockdown, as though this were some kind of raid on the compound. This guy just struck her as too cool and too eager to please. She wondered what he was up to.

"We'll need appropriate personnel with unrestricted access, but other than that your people can leave as scheduled," Kat said.

DeAngelo got on the phone and told someone on the other end to make an announcement that employees not involved in the inspection were free to leave.

"What now?" he asked cheerfully.

Even guys Kat knew full well weren't doing anything wrong were worried when the FDA showed up at their door. DeAngelo was playing by some alternative set of rules.

"I'm going to need all of your logs and financials. You have an office where I can work?" she asked.

He led her down a hallway and to a large office at the end. On the wall outside was a small, brass sign engraved with the name, Colton Barnes. She paused before entering. The office stood in stark contrast with the other standard issue offices she passed. This office was enormous, regal, and richly decorated with loads of mahogany and rich leather. It must have been her imagination, but as Kat entered, she thought she felt a distinct chill come over here, almost like a generalized feeling that the walls of this room held ominous secrets. Why DeAngelo would place her in his partner's office rather than opting for a conference room? Either he was trying too hard to prove that he was ignorant of what Barnes was up to right under his nose or it was a gesture of supreme arrogance. Kat inspected the room while she waited for DeAngelo to bring her the logs and lot testing records.

She was struck by the fact that the office, though beautiful, was starkly impersonal. She would have expected to see some football memorabilia, surely a picture of Barnes with his famous father, maybe even something from Penn. It was as though the office were done by a designer and all the "homey" touches were just for visual appeal and carried no personal significance. The only photo in the room was of Barnes standing with another guy holding a photo of an orchid.

DeAngelo returned with an armful of binders and plopped them on the enormous mahogany desk in front of Kat. She took a seat on the guest side of the desk, choosing not to be presumptuous as to make herself at home in Colton's leather desk chair. After DeAngelo laid down the binders, he turned and walked toward the door. Kat flipped open one of the binders and set her legal pad next to it, ready to take notes. Instead of exiting, DeAngelo closed the door and took up a seat across from Kat. She looked up at him, about to let him know that he needn't sit and wait with her, but before she could, he quietly spoke.

"I'll tell you everything," he said.

Chapter 9

Headline story, ABC, CBS, NBC, CNN, FOX, PBS, BBC:

...The incidences of tainted drugs in the United States prescription medication supply appears to have reached epidemic proportions, rapidly heading toward a pandemic. Counterfeits have been discovered in all of the top prescribed medications and in virtually every dosage form. Thousands of patients have been sickened and hundreds have died from allergic reactions. The death toll among patients whose diseases remain unmedicated is so far untallied...

***

"Guy swears there's another set of books on a separate computer," Kat announced to Lonny and Tyrell.

Kat was suspicious of DeAngelo's motives for telling them everything before they even asked. . He didn't seem like the kind of guy who was easily spooked. There had to be a story behind why he was so anxious to turn state's witness.

"Where?" Tyrell asked.

"Probably with Barnes, but DeAngelo says he's got the data on a flash drive," said Kat.

"Not sure I'd trust that. Can't verify the source," said Tyrell.

"You know my daddy had a saying: be cautious by one donkey calling another one 'long ears,'" offered Lonny.

Tyrell took a double take at Lonny, shook his head and asked, "What's he want?"

"Says he wants complete immunity," answered Kat.

"Why's he need it?" asked Lonny.

"That's what we have to find out," answered Kat.

"No deals before you see what he's got, right?" declared Tyrell, slapping his hand on the desk.

"She's not an idiot," Lonny shot back.

"Not sayin' that. Just thinkin'—"

"I'm going to take a look at the data. Meantime, I still want you two to brief the others and get them going over this place with a fine-toothed comb," said Kat.

Kat led the way to the door and down to the lobby where they met with the other investigators. Tyrell and Lonny held a short conference with each team, bringing them up to speed on the new information and asking them to conduct a second search concentrating on uncovering evidence of tampering and counterfeits. Kat waited for the investigators to leave and Tyrell and Lonny to rejoin her and DeAngelo, and then led the way back to Barnes' office.

"You're not going to find anything here," said DeAngelo as they made their way down the hallway.

"We'll decide that," countered Kat, without missing a beat.

"I'll tell you where you can find his operation," said DeAngelo.

"We'll have plenty of time for that, Mr. DeAngelo. Right now my team and I want to move through at our own pace," said Kat.

"Fine. But he's flying back into town now and I guarantee he'll have all of his people sewn up if you don't move fast enough. You want to make a case or not?" asked DeAngelo.

Kat stopped first. The others followed suit. She eyed DeAngelo for a long time. Something about his demeanor didn't sit quite right; he seemed too cocky about turning in his partner, too eager to get rid of the guy. Kat had to wonder whether DeAngelo was up to something. She glanced at Tyrell's face and saw that he shared her suspicions, and she trusted his barometer. Kat pointed at Tyrell and mouthed "you take it" as she let the way to Barnes' office. He nodded and gave her a thumbs-up.

Once they were settled, Tyrell sidled up to DeAngelo, looked him over and casually sat down on Colton's desk. He took a long pause to study him in silence. Finally, with an air of feigned disinterest, Tyrell began to speak.

"So, what's your angle, man? Thought this guy was a friend of yours. Isn't that why you partnered up in business?" Tyrell asked.

"My dad founded this business. He might have had his problems but he ran a decent business," said Jackie.

"But you're tellin' us this guy's dirty. So, how'd he get mixed up with him?" Tyrell asked.

"We were at Penn together—"

"Now, hold on there. You two were preppie college boys together, little frat boys?" Lonny chimed in.

The three exchanged glances. Kat knew the others were thinking what she was: if you knew this guy in college, you knew he was a drug lord, or at least every one else did. So, why go into business with him?

"We were roommates," Jackie explained.

"Didn't you know what his, ah, *business* was in college?" asked Tyrell. He leaned in closer to DeAngelo and looked him straight in the eye.

"The drug dealing? Yeah, everybody knew," said DeAngelo.

"I'm just an old country boy, but I'm having a hard time believing that you wanted to protect your daddy's business by partnering up with a *street* drug dealer," said Lonny.

"We needed a financial bailout. My dad had racked up gambling debts. I tried to cover him for years, but this time he'd gotten into them pretty bad. There was a hit out_"

"Ah, now, *you serious* with that? Hit men? What's all that bullshit," Tyrell shot.

Jackie showed just a hint of worry on his face that Kat picked up on immediately. Experience taught her that it was easier to get the truth out of a guy who absolutely believed he needed to tell the truth than a guy who knew they were using him to get to the real bad guy.

"He bought the business right out from under me! It was mine, my inheritance! I was entitled to it, not Colton Barnes. We just wanted a bailout, not a buyout!" DeAngelo raged.

The three watched as DeAngelo seemed to melt down in front of them, seemed to reveal his innermost motives, and seemed to be telling the truth. Kat knew better than to trust the display.

"Where're the financials?" she abruptly asked.

DeAngelo looked startled and Kat watched closely to see whether it was that he was having a genuine time moving away from his emotions or just angry that his acting wasn't as good as he thought it was.

"I— I got the data in my office," he answered.

She wanted to get a look at the data and decide for herself whether this guy as on the up and up. The data would be helpful, but if she got her hands on the actual computer with the data she'd be more convincing in court. Right now, just wanted to see if there was anything to DeAngelo's story.

"Go with him and get it," Kat directed Tyrell.

Tyrell led DeAngelo out of the room while Lonny stayed back. She paced the room a bit, and then abruptly turned to Lonny.

"How're you figuring this guy?" Kat asked.

"So far he seems like he's genuine, but you can never quite tell whether a dog's a pet or a wolf until there's fresh meat," offered Lonny.

Kat had to chuckle at Lonny's unique way of making a point. He was right. She'd have to reserve judgment until she saw the figures and heard what else he had to say. A minute later Tyrell returned with DeAngelo, who handed a flash drive to Kat before resuming his seat. Kat rounded the desk and popped the drive into Colton's desktop and opened the file. Lonny, Tyrell, and DeAngelo joined her behind the desk, waiting for the data to come up on the screen.

Once the numbers appeared, Kat felt like the room shifted rapidly sideways before the floor fell out from under. She steadied herself by clenching the arms of the chair. The numbers were staggering, shocking, and far more frightening than she imagined— maybe ten times what she thought they were up against. She felt sick to her stomach. If these were real, it was likely that hundreds of thousands of people might still be affected, with hundreds of thousands of innocent lives damaged or lost. And, for what? The stories and the faces rushed back and haunted her. She blinked them back and tried to keep them away from. But the more she did, the more her heart thumped in her chest. She turned and looked at Lonny and Tyrell, while attempting to remain cool and collected. She could tell by their faces that the numbers weighed on them too.

"Show us where the operation is," Kat croaked out.

"It's not here," Jackie answered and something in Tyrell snapped.

He reached out and grabbed Jackie around the neck and slammed him up against the wall with his full weight, his forearm pressing hard against Jackie's throat. It was no easy feat for a guy who was easily half DeAngelo's weight.

"You ain't in no position to play with us, you got that?!" Tyrell screamed.

Kat and Lonny quickly intervened. Kat grabbed Tyrell's arm to get him to relax his grip while Lonny talked him down with his "good ole boy" act. It didn't take long for the two of them to remove Tyrell from DeAngelo and get him over to the other side of the desk. Kat composed herself before approaching DeAngelo.

"Okay, let's try this again. Where's the operation?" she asked.

"There's a place over in Jersey that he's using. He has the counterfeit stuff trucked directly there, mixes with legitimate supply from here, fills orders and moves everything out," said DeAngelo.

"Where's supply coming from?" Kat asked.

"He's got a plant in India," Jackie replied.

Kat looked at Tyrell and Lonny. She decided on the spot that she and Tyrell were taking a road trip with DeAngelo while Lonny stayed behind and supervised the rest of the investigators.

"Tyrell, round up another five guys to go with us to Jersey," said Kat.

Tyrell left the room, then Kat pulled the flash drive and shoved it into her case.

"Where's Barnes now?" she asked DeAngelo.

"He's on his way back from St. Bart's. Should be landing in the next hour or so."

"Vacation?" she asked.

"Business," he replied.

"Deals on the counterfeits?" Kat asked.

"He knows better than to have a lot of cash hanging around, so he distributes it," Jackie said.

"Some kind of charity?" Kat asked.

"More like terrorists," Jackie casually said.

Kat held on to the edge of the desk. The room began to spin after DeAngelo's words. As if this guy weren't some kind of evil personified by tainting the prescription drug supply, now he was supporting terrorists? It was almost too awful to absorb.

"You're joking, right?" she shot back.

"Wish I were. He got onto this idea when all the money started rolling in. He said he wasn't going to get caught with all the extra cash like the stupid mob boys. He did all the usual stuff—offshore accounts, offshore real estate, anything that would use up the money. But I guess he got bored or something and started hosting audiences with terrorist groups in St. Bart's and giving money away. He gets off on it," Jackie said.

If it was true, maybe this DeAngelo really had reached his limit with Barnes. Maybe this was his shot to clear his conscience. The whole terrorist angle was something for the FBI and CIA boys to tackle. Kat's job was to identify the counterfeit sources and shut that operation down ASAP. The more she learned about this Colton Barnes, the more astonished she was by his blatant arrogance. A guy like that trumped Klein, and his fall was going to be a hard one.

"He know we're here?" Kat asked.

DeAngelo nodded. Kat contemplated her next move.

"Stall him when he calls next. Keep him out of here until tomorrow. Can you do that?"

"I can try," he said.

"Do more than try," added Lonny.

Tyrell returned to say that he had informed five of the agents that they were accompanying him to another site while the rest of the agents remained at his location under Lonny's supervision. Tyrell took DeAngelo out to the car, while Kat stayed behind to talk to Lonny.

"Use some of your small town charm and get some of these people to talk. I'm still having a hard time believing that all this was going on under their noses and no one got wind of it," she said.

"You think we need some police boys in case this Barnes fellow shows up?" Lonny asked.

"I don't want to bring those guys in just yet. If we don't have to spook Barnes, let's not. He shouldn't be surprised at our being here, but cops are another story," she replied.

"You want to leave me a copy of that data to look over, right?" Lonny asked.

Kat paused. It hit her that Lonny was not really asking for a copy of the data to examine, but a copy to have… just in case. She hadn't even considered that her road trip with DeAngelo could be dangerous. She winked at him and rummaged through her bag for a flash drive, sat down and copied all the data. When it was done, she handed it to Lonny and replaced the original in her bag.

As they were leaving the facility, a skinny guy wearing ugly glasses and holding a digital recorder loped toward them. Kat knew he had to be press. They tried to hurry and avoid the guy, but he called out to DeAngelo.

"Hey, Jackie. What's going on? I've been calling you for the past hour, but you're not picking up," the guy said.

"Hey, Rubano. Kind of busy now," Jackie replied.

"I can see that. Didn't I see you at the Jefferson summit? Talking to Colton? You FDA?" he asked Kat directly.

Kat glanced at DeAngelo, and then back to Rubano. She continued on toward the car, ignoring the reporter and trying to act as though everything was standard operating procedure. Of course, she didn't presume that he would buy that a bunch of FDA agents with the owner of a distributorship was the least bit ordinary, but she knew better than to utter so much as one word to a reporter. Kat, Tyrell, and DeAngelo got into one car, with the rest of the agents getting in the other. Rubano raced to his car and fired up. He was going to try to follow them.

"North or South Jersey?" she barked at DeAngelo.

"South," came the answer.

"What bridge?" she asked.

"Take the Barry," said Jackie.

Kat told Tyrell to call the agents in the other car and let them know they were trying to shake the reporter by taking the Schuylkill Expressway and looping around to I-95 to the Commodore Barry Bridge. Kat sped out of the parking lot, and cut across three lanes of traffic to get on the Expressway. She checked the rear view and saw that the other car of agents had kept up fine. She didn't see Rubano's car. She hoped she had shaken him off.

It took less than an hour to get to the warehouse just off I-295 in Salem County where DeAngelo led them to a nondescript building visible from the freeway, but only accessible by navigating a labyrinth of two-lane country roads. When they finally arrived at the South Jersey warehouse, Kat pulled around back to the loading dock and parked the car. The other agents were close behind.

"Anyone in there now?" Kat asked DeAngelo as she cut off the engine.

"Shouldn't be. They don't work after hours. Work regular day shift like any other business," he replied.

"How many employees?" Kat asked.

"About ten. One supervisor, one warehouse guy, and the rest are workers who do the actually mixing. They're all illegals except for the supervisor and warehouse guy," said Jackie.

"You got names?" Kat asked.

"Of course," Jackie replied.

Kat got out of the car and gave the game plan to the agents in the other car. She motioned for Tyrell to bring DeAngelo over to the rest of them in the parking lot.

"We're going inside to collect samples and document the place. Tyrell will hand out the assignments," said Kat.

While Tyrell broke up the other agents into teams, Kat walked DeAngelo to the back door of the facility and told him to open up. He fumbled around with a ring of multiple keys until he finally found the correct one and got the door open. She followed him inside, and stood in amazement after he flipped on the lights.

The warehouse was nondescript, just a big metal box with a few storage racks, no climate control, no ventilation control, and no sterility. The place could have been an ordinary warehouse holding any manner of goods:

TVs, refrigerators, furniture, bulk canned goods, auto parts, whatever. But it was not at all appropriate for handling solid dosage forms of life-saving prescription medications. There were standard issue cardboard barrels lined with plastic that held the various solid dosage forms that were being cleared through. There was no evidence of gloves, sterile suits, hair coverings, or anything that would indicate that precautions were taken to even ensure that rodents or other vermin didn't visit the various barrels of drugs. Kat had an odd thought, one that almost made her chuckle, because the first thing that came to mind was that this warehouse was in no way certified for sterility—and then she remembered what the goods inside were.

***

By the time Colton got to Philadelphia, he was hours behind schedule. Takeoff from St. Bart's was delayed, thanks to an on-board brawl between a pregnant woman and an older man that required intervention from local police. Colton had been calling Jackie since they landed, but only got him to answer the first time when he whispered that he couldn't talk. He left numerous voice mails, hoping that Jackie would at least pick them up and listen to his instructions, but he couldn't be sure, so he kept calling. As the plane moved to the gate, Jackie finally answered his phone.

"Everything's fine. They're out of here now," he said.

Colton checked his watch; it was ten o'clock. The FDA investigators had spent the last five hours crawling around his facility. When he thought about how the FDA's investigation had been brought about by the carelessness of the Chinese, he itched to personally kill each and every one of them. He had to take a deep breath and calm down. Though he was supremely confident the FDA wouldn't find anything out of the ordinary, he still worried that Jackie would say just one stupid thing that would trigger additional investigations.

"They coming back?" Colton asked.

"Tomorrow but didn't say when," Jackie replied.

"I'll be up there in about an hour," Colton said.

"No, no. Stay away. It would look bad if you suddenly showed up," Jackie said.

"It's my fucking company. I can come and go as I please, right? Why would that be suspicious?" Colton asked.

He suspected the real reason Jackie didn't want him up there was because he wanted to go home and sleep.

"Shit. One of them is coming back," said Jackie.

"Which one?" Colton asked.

"The woman. Vasquez," Jackie replied.

Colton didn't believe Jackie.

"Don't hang up. Let me hear you talk to her," he said.

"Colton—"

"Do it!"

Colton could hear the phone being jostled around and then a clunk as it was plopped down somewhere. At first he could only hear background noise, and then he heard Jackie talking and a woman's voice. He could not make out exactly what they were saying. He continued to listen as he walked off the plane and toward the airport parking lot. There was silence and finally Jackie came back on.

"You hear that? She wants to look at more of the log books," said Jackie.

"Now?" Colton asked, glancing at his watch.

"Probably some kind of technique they're using. I'm not arguing with her. I'm just handing them over," said Jackie.

"Shit! Let me know when she leaves. I'll be in first thing in the morning," said Colton.

He had made it all the way to the exit without realizing he was there or that Reggie was still by his side. He was jumpy, anxious to show up at the facility, but he knew it was too risky. He tossed around his next move, and then noticed Reggie next to him.

"Why you just standing here? Get up there and bring the car around!" he barked.

Reggie got him back to the condo in record time, but Colton really didn't want to be back at the condo. He hated this feeling of helplessness, hated to be at the mercy of anyone else. He expected to find Cherie asleep in bed, but when he entered, he found her sitting in the living room sharing tea with the Palestinian from St. Bart's. She was talking from the moment he entered, but Colton wasn't listening, instead he took a moment to survey the room, and then calculated how long it would take to get from the door to the bedroom night stand where he kept a loaded 9mm Glock.

He dropped his bag by the door and walked directly into the bedroom where he retrieved the Glock, checked the clip, cocked it, and then slowly walked back into the living room with the gun clearly visible at his side. With his other hand, he hit speed dial for Reggie. Cherie sat with her back to the hallway door, but the Palestinian had a clear view of Colton and the gun as he entered. The Palestinian stayed exactly where he was, and showed no signs of nervousness, no sign of a weapon of his own.

"How the fuck did you find me?" Colton said.

Cherie stiffened and whipped around to look at Colton. At first her face was pinched in anger, but when she saw the gun, she changed to terror.

"Cherie, get in the bedroom and close the door," Colton said.

She bolted from the couch and rushed into the bedroom, just as Colton got through to Reggie.

"Get over here, now!" he yelled. He stashed the phone in his pocket. Through all, the Palestinian never moved, never even flinched.

"I was sharing with your lovely fiancé here—" he began.

"Get out." Colton growled.

"There is no need to fear me. You are the very best of a friend."

Colton took a step closer and aimed the gun at the Palestinian's head.

"One more time: how did you find me?" he asked.

The Palestinian rose from his seat and began repeatedly bowing. Colton kept the gun poised on the man's forehead and followed it as he bobbed up and down.

"I am your servant. I come to offer my deep, deep gratitude for all that you have done. When I heard of your engagement, I came to offer you congratulations," the Palestinian said.

Then, seemingly from nowhere, he produced a gold box and held it in his outstretched hands. He bowed his head low, so low that he could not have seen if Colton had decided to pull the trigger. Once again, Colton ignored his instincts and allowed himself to be intrigued by this man and touched by the gift. Even with a gun aimed at his head, the man showed no signs of fear. Colton reached out and retrieved the box. He ordered the Palestinian to sit back down in the chair and he glanced at the box.

"I am good at what I do, yes?" the man said.

Colton wasn't sure whether the man referred to the gold work or the fact that he found where Colton lived. He regarded the gold box in his hand again and it suddenly occurred to him that it might be rigged to explode, so he tossed it back into the Palestinian's lap and ordered him to open it. The man did so with a smile. He turned the box around to reveal the contents: a solid gold Rolex watch ringed with a band of diamonds set around the bezel. Colton reached out and took the box from the Palestinian and examined it more closely.

"Your mother didn't make this," Colton said.

The man chuckled. "No, no. The watch is a Rolex. My mother made the box."

Colton closed the box and looked at the top. There were intricate patterns carved into the gold and around the carvings was an oval of small, colorful gemstones. On the outside of the ring of gems there were more intricate carvings in the gold. Just as Colton finished studying the box, he heard the key in the front door lock and seconds later Reggie burst in and charged at the Palestinian, gun drawn, shouting, "Hands in the air!" In one swift motion Reggie jammed the gun into to the man's temple and wrapped his arm around his neck from behind. Once Reggie had secured him, Colton lowered his gun and sat down on the couch where he examined the watch and box more closely.

"Once again, your mother is supremely talented. More sacred gold?" Colton asked.

The Palestinian grinned and nodded furiously. He seemed to enjoy the joke of the sacred gold as much as Colton.

"So, how did you find me?" Colton asked, this time locking eyes with the man.

"As I said, I am very good at everything I do. On Saturday, I found the Prime Minister of Israel," he replied, referring to the assassination attempt on the life of the Prime Minister of Israel while he was vacationing in an undisclosed location.

Colton acknowledged the man's prowess with a tip of his head. The man smiled in return. Colton knew now that he needed to post an armed guard outside his door.

"Thanks for the gift. Reggie, take the man down to the street and get him a cab," he said.

"Many, many thanks. To you I am a friend," the Palestinian said as Reggie escorted him out of the condo.

After they were gone, Colton heaved a sigh of relief and sat on the couch waiting for his heart rate to return to normal. Then he went to the bedroom to retrieve Cherie. She was huddled in corner of the bed furthest away from the door, covers tight around her neck, and her knees pulled up to her chest. She was rocking like a child.

"You okay?" he asked.

"Mmmmm. Not so sure," she replied.

Colton sat down beside her and stroked her arm. For the first time he thought about what it would be like to lose her. He leaned over and wrapped his arms around her.

"Why did you let him in?" he asked.

"I remembered him from St. Bart's. He asked if he could wait for you. I didn't want to offend him…"

"Cherie, you have to get smarter about this kind of stuff. These guys—"

She drew back from him and got up on her knees.

"Colton, how would I know any better? I didn't even know where you were or what time you were coming home. If you don't want me to make mistakes, then don't set me up for them!"

Annoyed by her tone, Colton got up and headed out the door, saying "Not now, Cherie. I need a drink."

He exited the room and went to the bar where he poured a stiff drink and sat down on the coach with his drink. In another moment, Cherie appeared.

"So who the hell was that really? I'm entitled to an answer," she demanded.

"You tell me. Seems like you made best of friends with the guy," he shot back.

"He told me he was an associate of yours, a Mr. Hamon," she said.

"So you just invited the guy in and made tea? It's the middle of the fucking night! Are you stupid?" Colton shouted.

She stared at him without reply.

"That was unnecessary. And by the way, where the hell were you?" she asked.

Colton stifled the impulse to clock her one across the face. He had enough problems without creating more. He took a long drink to calm himself before he replied.

"My plane was stuck on the runway," he said.

"Your plane!? You just take off and don't tell me where you are? Is that how it's going to be?" she screamed.

"Yes, that's how it's going to be," he replied.

He slammed his glass down on the counter. Cherie flinched, but then hitched one hip and crossed her arms in front of her chest.

"We had an appointment that you missed," she jabbed.

"Fuck your appointments!" he screamed back.

She drew back. After some moments, she spoke in a soft tone.

"Colton—"

"Not one more word, Cherie," he said. "Not one."

He expected more words from her, but when he looked up, he saw how her face had softened. She looked scared and hurt and sad.

"I'm sorry, honey," she whimpered. "I was worried about you and I thought it was okay with Mr. Hamon and then the gun... I was just so scared…"

Tears streamed down her face and he hesitated. Then he stepped over to her and enveloped her in a tight embrace. He was surprised at how good it felt to hold her and how awful it would be to lose her. They stood together until her sobbing quieted.

"Why don't you try to get some sleep?" he said finally.

She loosened up her grip and took a step back from him, looked into his eyes.

"Do you love me?" she asked.

The question caught him off guard.

"Of course," he stammered, surprising himself at his sincerity.

"I really do love you," she said. "You can trust that. Then she padded toward the bedroom and quietly closed the door.

He didn't know what to say to her. He was still angry, but he was beginning to feel about her the way he had never felt about anyone else in his life. That scared him about as much as the thought of losing her. He was about to follow her when Reggie called.

"Where'd he go?" Colton asked.

"I dropped him in North Philly. Figure he'll have some kind of time getting out of there alive, huh?" Reggie snickered.

"I need protection here 24/7," said Colton.

"Tonight?" Reggie replied.

"Yeah, tonight! What the fuck else did you think 24/7 meant?" Colton barked.

He tapped the phone off and tossed it on the couch. He was trying to channel the anger simmering inside of him, control the feeling that too much debris was crashing down around him. He wished he had killed Ho with his own hands; he could have used that feeling right now. He should have known better. He should not have been deceived by the Palestinian's apparent good will. He felt betrayed. He treated people well and yet they hurt him, took advantage of him. Every one of his best efforts was thwarted by someone putting their own wants and needs ahead of his.

He sat on the couch in the dark, staring out the window at the Kammerly Center, trying to stop the continuous list of slights from running through his mind, from driving him to hate. His eyes traced the shapes of the glass atrium on the rooftop, contemplating his next move. He hated that he couldn't shut down Kat Vasquez and the FDA with a single bullet, hated that he needed Cherie, hated that the Palestinian was cleverer than he, and most especially hated that he was not treated with the respect that he deserved.

He walked over to the custom-built glass shelving next to the window, the home of his precious orchids. Not long after he and Cherie moved into the condo, he noticed the perfect amount of eastern light that shone in through the front, right to the side of the floor-to-ceiling plate glass window. It was the perfect kind of light for his darlings. The sun's warmth caressed his prized possessions; the thickness of the noise abatement glass protected them from the winter chill.

Being with his collection soothed him and calmed the thoughts racing through his mind. He caressed the silken petals of his phalaenopsis amabilis, his first orchid, bought at the Philadelphia Flower Show and lovingly transported home and given a place of honor in the kitchen of his old brick row home. It thrived there, happy under Colton's hovering care and the light from the back window.

"What the fuck's this?" his father had asked.

Daddy had just come from scouting talent and surprised Colton by showing up on his doorstep, something the famous coach had never done. Colton had tried to put him off, suggesting they go out and grab a couple of beers somewhere, but Daddy had pushed his way in and headed straight for the refrigerator where he downed his first beer almost before Colton could even catch up with him. He had grabbed a second can and hovered in the kitchen drinking. That's when he had spotted the orchid.

"It's a phalaenopsis amabilis," Colton said proudly.

"A faggoty what, what?" said Daddy.

"It's an orchid," Colton replied.

"Some girlie get that for you, or you get it yourself, twinkle toes?" his father said.

"So how are the prospects looking this year?" Colton said, hoping that changing the subject would diffuse his father. But once Daddy got stuck on something, he was stuck for good.

"What do you care? Seems like you'd rather be a fruity decorator than talk about football," he replied.

"So is Drake healed up from his injury? Ready to go back to being the quarterback in the league?" Colton persisted.

He had desperately fished for something to say that would reprogram Daddy and get him off the subject of the orchid.

"I don't like this fairy looking thing," Daddy had declared, and then grabbed the bloom-covered stem, snapped it off, tossed it on the floor and ground it into the hardwood with his filthy Nike. He knocked the pot onto the floor and stomped on the plant for good measure. Daddy downed his second beer, slammed the can on the counter and headed for the door. "At least try to be a man like your brother," he had said just before he slammed the door shut.

For the next six months, Colton had nursed his plant back to health. Finally, it had bloomed again, more magnificently than before, thriving under his tender care. Since then it had enjoyed an honored place among his collection. Colton stroked the leaves, gazed at the pure, white petals that seemed to glow in the moonlight and felt calmed, proud of how he saved his cherished friend. He surveyed the rest of his plants, reciting their names and descriptions like a prayer: Phaiocalanthe Kryptonite or chariot of fire, a vivid, rich burgundy color with a pink and white center; Laelia purpurata, white with pink lip, lovely, graceful; Cattleya amethystoglossa. a large, classic orchids; Milt. Celle "Hinsdale", a deep red with a firework splotch of white and a center of deep yellow; and Dendrobium Spring Dream "Kumiko", a cluster of white gems riotously arranged on a stem with deep, green leaves. Each one lovingly cared for, each rare specimen rewarded him for his care and attention, and each one never disappointed him. He carefully checked the moisture level of each plant, touching the roots and the stems, gauging each one's needs. He picked up the water bottle and gingerly misted only the plants in need, taking care not to offer too much moisture, opening the opportunity for rot. Satisfied with his handiwork, he stepped back and admired his collection, studying each velvety bloom, each sprinkling of color, and each magnificent shape. Benoit came to mind.

"Reggie," he barked into his phone.

"Boss?" Reggie replied, voice hoarse from sleep.

"You outside my door?" Colton asked.

"Yeah," Reggie replied.

"It's not helping me if you're asleep," Colton said.

"Sorry, Boss."

"The caretaker at the St. Bart's villa, a guy named Benoit. He's going to bring me something. Arrange for him to fly up here and deliver it to me tomorrow," said Colton.

"You sure that's a good idea these days? Maybe you should—"

"Maybe everyone around me needs to shut the fuck up and do what I say!" Colton barked.

He hung up the phone and stomped around the condo, frustrated and angry again. All the calmness of the last half hour with his beloved orchids had disappeared. He gulped down another drink, feeling the liquid burn his throat, happy to know that the alcohol would soon take the edge off.

He retreated to the study and rummaged in the back of the closet where he had stashed the work laptop. While he waited for the laptop to get fully on-line, he retreated back to the bar and poured another drink. The screen came alive and Colton clicked on a file folder marked Orchid Collection I, typed in the password, and watched as the spreadsheet of his entire business appeared before him. The numbers were impressive, by any standards. They reminded him of his own cleverness and calmed him. He opened the Orchid Collection file and perused the numbers, mentally calculating the difference between the real USA money and the money that Uncle Sam and all the others, save for Hugh, thought USA was making. Then he checked the list of manufacturers and calculated shipment dates, mentally charting his supplier shipments when the issues began. The Chinese plant supplied most of his inventory, but the numbers from the Manchester plant were only about 30 percent lower than the Chinese production. He would have to plan a trip to England in the next couple of weeks.

Colton studied the spreadsheets, production numbers and ratios, margins, and every conceivable number he could commit to memory. The numbers were like a soothing mantra.

***

In the Office of Criminal Investigations interrogation room, Jackie told OCI head Paul Thuyen everything he wanted to hear, but he didn't tell him the truth. None of Colton's players would ever know that Jackie was responsible for his disappearance. Most of them would only briefly care that Colton was gone because they would know that after Colton, there was still Jackie and there was still good money.

"Is there anything you have to add to your statement, Mr. DeAngelo?" the investigator asked.

"That's everything," answered Jackie.

"If you hear from Mr. Barnes, let us know."

"Absolutely," Jackie assured him. "We appreciate your cooperation."

Thuyen escorted Jackie out of the room and down the hall to the exit. They shook hands and Jackie exited the building.

He felt the cool night air on his face and stifled his impulse to snicker. As he wove through the cars to his own, Rubano was coming right at him and so he quickened his pace.

"Jackie! C'mon, talk to me. I already know Colton was involved, but I'll give you a chance to tell your side of the story," he called.

Jackie hurried to get inside his car, but Rubano caught the door before Jackie could close it.

"Just tell me where Colton is. I'll talk to him," Rubano said.

"Nobody's gonna talk to you, Rubano," Jackie said.

He yanked on the door, but the reporter had a good hold of it and it stayed open.

"C'mon, you know me. You know I'll be fair. Just tell me your side of the story," Rubano pleaded.

"You want a story? Find Colton," said Jackie.

He pushed Rubano away and managed to get the door closed and locked. He started up the engine and pulled away as Rubano scrambled back to his car to follow. Jackie took a number of extra turns until he knew for sure that

Rubano had lost him, and then made his way home. He pulled into the garage, shut the engine and the garage door and sat in the dark. At first he held his face impassive. Then he began to laugh out loud.

It was almost midnight by the time he made his way into the house. Donna and the kids were already in bed. He paced through the house, opening and closing doors, entering and leaving rooms, trying to work off his nervous energy. He grabbed a quick snack from the fridge, fussed over the mail and mindlessly wiped the fingerprints off the refrigerator door with a wad of paper towels. He resisted the temptation to call Hamon. He tried to tamp down his curiosity about what he had done with Colton and the girl. Finally, he plopped himself on the family room recliner, flipped on the television, scanned the channels and finally stopped on a documentary on the construction of wind turbines. He forced himself to watch until finally he felt his eyes droop and his head bob. He switched off the television and crawled into bed with Donna and fell asleep.

***

Kat spent the morning conferring with Paul Thuyen, head of the FDA's regional Office of Criminal Investigations at his office in downtown Philadelphia. While she was there, she instructed Jackie to lure Barnes to USA Distributors and act as though nothing were out of the ordinary, buying time while she waited for Thuyen to obtain a warrant to search Barnes' condo. The last thing she wanted was a premature confrontation with Barnes. All evidence seemed to indicate he was violent. Her hope was that the laptop containing the real data was still in the condo, as well as other items of interest. Thuyen was waiting for the judge to issue the warrant. Kat paced the office, pretending to patiently wait with him.

"Any ETA?" Kat asked for the umpteenth time.

"It'll be here soon," Thuyen answered flatly.

Kat returned to her pacing, but then left the office and wandered down the hallway, desperately trying to walk off her nervous energy. She was beginning to complete calculations in her head on the amount of drug that Barnes had already put out into the marketplace and how much might be left in the pipeline. Any way she calculated, the numbers were still staggering. The only bright spot was that, according to DeAngelo, Barnes was spooked off enough to temporarily shut down the counterfeit operation. Now the FDA would be in the awkward position of negotiating with the drug manufacturers to increase production to meet increased demand, as well as devote additional resources to make sure lots got out of quarantine and to market in half the time. And, all of it had to take place under the watchful eye of Kneeley and the committee. The Senator added to the pressure by insisting that he should make the announcement of the arrest to the public and take all the credit for saving the American drug supply.

"Kat, you know a guy named Rubano?" Thuyen said as he stuck his head out into the hallway.

"Why?" Kat asked.

"He's on my phone," Thuyen replied.

"Shit! How'd he get on to this? He could blow the whole thing!" she said.

"I'll get rid of him," he said.

Thuyen disappeared into this office and Kat continued to pace the hallway. Late the night before she had decided to pull in OCI, after she got verification from the labs at HQ that what came from the Jersey warehouse was adulterated in spite of being a perfect match in appearance to the real drug. Jackie had supplied them the names of the warehouse staff, most of them illegals who scattered once they got word that the authorities were onto the operation. Kat knew there was little hope of ever tracking them down again. But the guy DeAngelo said was in charge of the warehouse was "One Eye" Willy, a South Philly wise guy with loose mob connections who usually stuck to gambling and loan sharking operations. Jackie had handed her a sheaf of paperwork and emails that pretty much made their entire case against that guy and helped mount even more evidence against Barnes. Not long after her phone call to Thuyen, she got a call. Philadelphia police had arrested One Eye in Atlantic City.

"Okay, Judge Bollingbrooke signed the warrant. We're good to go," said Thuyen as he dashed by Kat on his way out the door. Kat scurried to catch up.

***

Colton hadn't spoken with Jackie since the night before and now his calls were going right into voice mail. It was only six o'clock in the morning, but Colton was anxious to get to his office and meet with these FDA jokers face-to-face. He was too antsy to wait for Reggie to pull the Escalade around, so he went with him to the underground parking garage. As he waited for Reggie to pull the truck out of the parking spot, he felt a hand around his arm.

"So, what's going on over there at USA Distributors?" asked Rubano.

Colton violently jerked his hand away as he realized it was Rubano. Reggie was out of the truck and on top of Rubano in a blink, wrestling him to the ground and shouting for him to get the hell away from Colton.

"They're crawling all over your business, Colton!" Rubano shouted. "It's something more than just routine. C'mon, let me tell your side of the story!"

"Stay the hell away from me!" Colton shot back.

"They got Jackie. You know that? Five, six investigators escorted him out of the building and stuffed him in the back of a car. I tried to follow them, but they lost me," Rubano said.

Colton tried to stay cool, but Rubano's words hit him like a sledgehammer.

"What did you see?" Colton walked closer to Rubano, who was still being held by Reggie.

"Must have been ten or more investigators there," he said.

"Cops?" Colton asked.

"Don't think so. I checked with local contacts and they haven't been pulled in. Strictly FDA at this point. OCI division too," Rubano said.

"Let him go, Reggie," said Colton.

Reggie hesitated, but Colton nodded his okay again and Reggie let go.

"You wanna talk? I'll give you an exclusive. Your side of the story," said Rubano as he scrambled to his feet.

"What makes you think I've got a story?" Colton asked.

"C'mon Colton. I've been tracking these guys since this story hit. One, maybe two investigators at a location, tops. You got more than ten. I can do the math," he said.

Colton signaled for Reggie to get back into the truck, and he followed, leaving Rubano all alone. Reggie took off fast up the ramp, pulling South on Broad and heading toward the freeway entrance. Colton tried to hold himself together, but as he ran Rubano's words around in his head, he clenched his jaw. Either these guys were on to him or Jackie had talked.

"You get hold of Jackie?" Colton suddenly asked.

"Still goes straight to voice mail," Reggie replied.

Colton tapped his iPhone and called Jackie again. This time the call was picked up. "Where the fuck have you been?"

"What? Sleeping. Jeez Colton, you scared me," said Jackie.

"I'm on my way to the office. Meet me there," said Colton.

"What time is it?" Jackie asked.

"It's time for you to fucking do your job right!" Colton screamed.

"What the fuck? Colton, I handled those guys just fine yesterday. We're good," Jackie replied.

"I don't know that! All I know is what you told me and that's not enough. I need to see for myself and you're going to show me! Now!" Colton barked.

"Okay, okay. I said I'd be there!" Jackie answered.

Colton tapped Jackie off the phone and punched the dashboard, almost breaking his hand. Rubano's words rattled around in Colton's head again. He needed to devise a way to test Jackie, to find out whether he got in bed with that damn Kat Vasquez or not. He called Rack at home.

"You guys get any visitors there yesterday?" he asked.

"Nope. No one," Rack replied.

There was no hint of hesitation in Rack's voice.

"Not even Jackie?" Colton probed.

"Nope. Everything's quiet. I saw on the news you got guys up at your place," Rack said.

"Yeah, they're all over everybody. Anyone new hanging around there, anybody you don't recognize?" Colton asked.

"Not at all. But I'll let you know if I see anything," Rack said.

Colton wanted to be reassured by what Rack said. He had always trusted Rack, but he still wondered about Jackie. Maybe Jackie had gotten to Rack too. Maybe everyone was plotting against him. He was frustrated, feeling like he was not the master of his own realm, unable to reassure himself that things were all right for fear of tipping off the FDA. It was too risky to visit the Jersey facility. He had no way to verify that Jackie had fixed things properly. Colton felt himself sweating through his shirt and wiped the moisture away from his top lip. To help calm himself down, he began to inventory of all the reasons why his set up was undetectable: the USA Distributors site was clean, all the operation was carried out off-site, the records were clean, all the records were in his possession, and the personnel, with the exception of Jackie, Reggie and Hugh, had no idea about the other operation. He heaved a faint sigh of relief. Then he ran down the insurance he had on each of his players, calculated maneuvers he had made just to make sure that his people stayed loyal: he paid for round-the-clock home health aides for Reggie's mom, covered up for Hugh's drunk driving accident when he clipped a pedestrian, and took good care of Stewart and Gus with extra cash. That left just Jackie. He may have bailed out his father's company, but that didn't necessarily buy Jackie's loyalty. In fact, it probably only bought Jackie's resentment. He needed something more direct to hold over Jackie.

"You hang out with Jackie, right?" he asked.

"Sometimes," Reggie replied.

"You ever seen him step out on Donna?" Colton asked.

Reggie burst out laughing.

"He tries to get away from that cunt all the time, but he's scared stiff. Can't even get it up he's so afraid she'll cut off his balls if she catches him," Reggie said.

Colton joined in the laughter, relishing the thought of Jackie with his nuts in a vise and his wife's hands on the grip. He might be able to work that angle, although he had hoped for something better. If he couldn't find anything to hold over Jackie, he would have to engineer it.

As he was mulling over his the problem, Reggie pulled into the parking lot. Colton spied Jackie's car near the entrance and that damn pesky Rubano pacing outside the front door. Reggie pulled up to the front door, almost hitting Rubano in the process. Colton jumped out of the truck and slipped into the building before Rubano had a chance to get near him.

He looked around the facility, half expecting a posse of investigators or maybe even FBI or cops to surround him, but the place was empty. And quiet. He peered down the hallway and saw the light on in Jackie's office and headed in that direction, pausing only slightly at each door along the way, searching for an imagined ambush. He found Jackie sitting at his desk, studying something on the screen in front of him.

"What the fuck's going on?!" Colton demanded.

Jackie looked up and frowned, and then leaned back in his chair as though it were any other casual morning.

"Everything's fine," Jackie said.

Colton stared at him for a long time, straight into his eyes, hoping to either intimidate him or see deeply enough to know whether Jackie was lying. Then it dawned on him that Jackie may be wired. Without another word, he reached across the desk and patted him down, looking for a device. Jackie complied without protest and after a thorough examination, Colton stepped away, satisfied that he was clean. He motioned for Jackie to follow him into the warehouse and waited until they were both there to speak.

"Vasquez and how many others?" Colton demanded.

"Ten. They went over the place, all routine stuff. Looked at the logs, went over the financials, checked with the managers… Nothing out of the ordinary," Jackie replied.

"You said yesterday that there were only two," said Colton.

"Yeah, yeah, at first. Then the rest of them showed up," Jackie replied.

Colton eyed Jackie carefully, watching, weighing.

"Why so many?" he asked.

"How the hell do I know? Extra pressure from Washington is my bet. Belvadere said he had about five go over his place and Jacobson said he had the same number. It's just the atmosphere. They're not on to anything, Colton. How could they be? You're just too smart for them," Jackie said, leaning back in his chair.

He eyed Jackie carefully, searching for a sign, any sign—beads of sweat, a nervous twitch, blinking eye—anything that would betray a lie. Jackie seemed like always: no more or less nervous, no more or less cooperative.

"Rubano said you took them someplace yesterday," Colton said.

"More like they took me down for interrogation," Jackie grumbled.

"Oh, interrogation, huh?" said Colton.

"You don't believe me? You think I took them to the warehouse? Call Rack. No, I'll call Rack myself." He grabbed his phone and tapped in Rack's number.

"Don't bother. I already talked to him," Colton answered.

Jackie hung up the phone and shoved it back into his pocket. Then he plopped down in his chair. "Jesus Colton! Do you think I'm fucking stupid?"

"Stupid or too smart. I'm not sure which. You just might find yourself a dead man, Jackie," Colton said.

Jackie stared at Colton, narrowed his eyes.

"You would do that? Just like that? We've spent almost our whole lives together, our whole lives, and you would throw it away just like that?" Jackie demanded.

Colton turned away from Jackie, unable to look him in the eye. He headed for the door, then paused, his back to Jackie.

"They coming back today?" he asked.

Jackie sighed deeply, and finally answered. "Probably. They already got all the samples they needed, but Vasquez wanted to go over the logs again."

Colton glanced at his iPhone for the time and retreated to his office without another word.

***

On the way to Barnes' condo, Kat checked in with Jackie.

"Is he there?" she asked.

"Yeah, he's here," Jackie replied.

"Make sure he stays there for at least two hours," said Kat.

The team stood outside the cars and mapped out the strategy for executing the warrant. After about ten minutes of putting the final touches on the plan, they made their way to the front doors of Symphony House where armed Philadelphia police officers greeted them.

The enlarged team had one last meeting outside Symphony House, and then the doorman ushered them into the elevator as the building manager stood in the lobby to intercept any press curiosity seekers who might show up. It was eerily silent in the elevator up. Kat reviewed the plan in her head and braced for what further revelations might be found in Colton Barnes' condo.

The police officers stood near the front door with weapons drawn. A female officer motioned for Thuyen and Kat to stay back near the elevator until the officers gave them the all clear to enter. The additional team members, two of Thuyen's officers and a computer specialist, huddled behind Thuyen and Kat, watching the officers try to gain entry into the condo. There was some previous discussion about whether the girlfriend would still be home. The female officer that now held them back from the door was assigned to handle the girlfriend if she were found at home.

First, the officers knocked on the door and announced themselves as police. No answer. They knocked a second time and identified themselves. No answer again. They signaled to one of Thuyen's people to radio the building managers that they needed passkeys to open the door. Then, they waited in silence. Kat could hear the elevator making its way to their floor and soon the building manager appeared with the key. One of the officers who had been standing at the condo door retrieved the key and opened the door. Two officers brandishing weapons shouted, "Police! Anyone home?", and then disappeared inside. Kat heard them continue to identify themselves as they moved around the condo, making sure it was secure before anyone else entered. Finally, after what seemed like an inordinate amount of time, one officer emerged and gave the all clear. Thuyen and his two guys took off immediately and Kat straggled behind.

She lingered in the living room of the condo while the others tore the place apart as they searched. Kat was only interested in the laptop and verifying the information she already had; the rest were searching for whatever else they could find that would help make the case against Colton Barnes. Like Barnes' office, the place was perfectly decorated, perfectly fashionable, and mostly sterile. She ventured over to the windows along the front of the condo, the ones that overlooked Broad Street and gave a view all the way down to the Delaware River. There was no doubt that a view like that would make a person feel powerful enough to think that ordinary rules didn't apply to them. She studied the meticulously kept orchids on their glass shelves, wondering whether they were the pride of Barnes or the girlfriend. Then she moved onto the grand piano positioned near the north windows in the corner so the atrium of the Kammerly Center served as the backdrop. Kat tried to grasp how much one human must hate that he would treat himself to such luxury yet murder so many others without so much as a second thought.

"Ah, Vasquez. We found a laptop," said one of Thuyen's men.

When Kat got to the office, the computer specialist had already booted up the laptop and placed it on the desk next to the desktop computer. He did an extensive diagnostics first, identifying which programs had been recently accessed and when, and then opened each of those files while Kat observed. There didn't seem to be anything of particular business importance on the desktop, so the technician moved on to the laptop.

Again, he ran the same diagnostics and proceeded to systematically open up files while Kat looked on. This time, the file appeared on the very first try. It was the last file Colton Barnes had opened late last night and kept open for a couple of hours. The specialist cracked the password in a matter of a minute and opened the file. The sight of those same numbers sent a chill down Kat's spine and the thought of Colton Barnes sitting in his multi-million dollar condo proudly pouring over the numbers from his reign of death made Kat nauseous. Jackie had indeed supplied them with a copy of the file; complete in all of its frightening details. The other FDA OCI agents also glanced at the numbers and gradually Kat heard the gasps and whistles of the agents as they first saw the numbers, then a pall descended over the entire room.

"We've got him," Kat said to Dan on the phone.

Chapter 10

Kat walked in on Tyrell and Lonny playing a game of one-on-one with crumpled papers and a corner trashcan in the OCI interrogation room. They snapped to attention immediately and pretended that they were having an important discussion.

"What's the score?" she asked.

The two looked at one another and snickered.

"Well, you know *I'm* winnin'," answered Tyrell.

"Not by much," countered Lonny.

Kat smiled, then plopped down into a chair and kicked off her shoes. Tyrell and Lonny took up seats across from her and waited.

"Thuyen's men, the local police, and the FBI are on their way to USA Distributors to pick up Barnes," she said evenly.

At first Tyrell and Lonny both nodded. Then Tyrell jumped out of his seat, whooping and hollering and doing a victory dance. Lonny slapped the table and smiled.

"The partner's story panned out. We've got the warehouse, the supplier, the equipment, falsified logs and testing, everything," she said.

"Dan's gotta be jumpin' like a toad on a hot skillet," said Lonny.

"You guys have earned some time off. You're on your own for the rest of the day and I'll see you back here tomorrow when we have a chance to talk to Mr. Barnes in person," said Kat.

"I'll be lookin' forward to that," said Tyrell.

Kat hung around the office awhile longer, debating whether to dive immediately into all the evidence. Instead, she went back to her hotel to change into clothes appropriate for a romping good time with Bernie. Chances were she would be up most of the night preparing for her interrogation of Barnes. Clearing her head now would make it easier to focus later.

Albe was in class when she arrived at the frat house, but the boys let her in. She piled Bernie into the truck for the short ride along Kelly Drive to the parking lot beside Penn boathouse. Her walk turned out to be more of a run; she struggled to keep a hold of Bernie as he chased a flock of fat geese hanging out on the riverbank. She enjoyed her jaunt almost as much as Bernie. The weather had turned a few degrees warmer and the river seemed still, tranquil. For the first time since the whole thing began, she was able to run hard, exhale all the fear and anger, and maybe finally stop the parade of dead and dying that marched toward her every time she closed her eyes. After running the length of Kelly Drive and back and working up a good sweat, she and Bernie collapsed in the back of the truck. She left the back gate open and sat next to him until they both caught their breath.

"The guys at your son's frat thought you'd be here," said Jimmy.

Kat instinctively smiled, then panicked. Jimmy was the last guy she should be talking to. She looked around, worried that someone would see them together.

"Get out of here, Jimmy," Kat said.

He stepped closer to the truck, which roused Bernie who stood at attention next to Kat and emitted a low growl. Kat kept a tight hold on his leash.

"The press is reporting that you guys are about to make a move on Barnes," he said.

"You know I can't talk to you, Jimmy," she replied.

It was agony to have to stay away from him. She tried not to look in his eyes, tried not to remember how grateful she was to him for pushing her to try love after Jorge. She caught a faint whiff of his smell and tried to ignore it. He stepped closer to her. Bernie snarled. Kat pushed the dog further into the truck and slammed the hatch closed. Jimmy tried to take her hand but she quickly pulled it away and shoved her hands into her pockets. He leaned into her and spoke softly.

"Kat, you've got the wrong idea. He called me in to talk a buyout. Remember how he approached me at the Kammerly? Said he wanted to talk?" Jimmy said.

Kat wanted to believe him and knew that she couldn't. She stepped back away from him, stumbled slightly, and then leaned on the truck.

"If you haven't done anything wrong, it'll come out. You have to believe that," she replied.

"C'mon Kat. It's me, Jimmy. You know me. You've known me for years. I'm not Barnes. What we had was real. Once this blows over, we'll be good. I'm asking for your help here."

Kat couldn't look at him. She didn't want to remember his face like this.

"Sorry, Jimmy," she said.

She brushed by him and got into the truck. She caught a look at his face in the mirror. He looked stunned and lost—nothing at all like the Jimmy Kirk she knew. The engine roared to life and Jimmy stayed right where she had left him, looking defeated. She drove off, watching him grow smaller and smaller in the mirror.

***

By two o'clock Colton was looking for a way to blow off steam. He'd been waiting for Kat Vasquez all day, and he took the hot shot FDA investigator's no-show to mean she wasn't all she was cracked up to be, that he'd designed an enterprise that was virtually undetectable. He smirked. He'd pulled his counterfeits off the market, forced the Chinese to lie low, and now he just needed to wait. After a few months, maybe as many as six, he'd start ramping the business up again and he'd be back to St. Bart's, back to being The Money Man. He knew now that neither the FDA nor Congress would be able to put anything in place that he couldn't maneuver around. He had to follow up with the Chinese, make sure they understood that what happened to Ho would happen to all of them unless they stayed out of his market. And he needed to deal with the Palestinian.

"Mr. Barnes, there's a Kristin for you on line one," said Betsy.

Colton picked up the phone, feeling his crotch stir.

"Colton Barnes," he said.

"Kristin from Atlantic City. Just wanted to let you know that I'm in the area this afternoon, Colton Barnes. You interested?" she purred.

Colton didn't hesitate.

"Meet me at the Valley Forge Hilton in half an hour," he said.

"Mmmmmm. How about Valley Forge *Park*?" she countered.

Colton frowned.

"Not really a nature kind of guy," he said.

"It'll be worth your while. I'll have a special surprise for you…" she sang.

Colton hesitated. He didn't feel like games, but he was intrigued.

"Make it worth my while," he finally said.

"Don't I always? Meet me in the parking lot off Valley Creek Road, where the Mount Misery trail begins," she said.

Colton hung up and sighed. He wasn't in the mood for games, but he knew Kristin was well worth it. She was the perfect antidote to the past few days. He pulled up a map of Valley Forge Park on-line, found the parking lot, and figured out his route. He stopped by Jackie's office on his way out.

"So where's this Vasquez?" he demanded.

Jackie looked up, startled, clicked his mouse, then leaned back in his chair and gave Colton his full attention.

"I guess they're done. I've been telling you everything went fine," he answered.

Colton studied Jackie's face, from the dark, receding eyes down to the second chin. He watched Jackie pick at the chewed nubs of his fingernails.

"You talk to some of the other guys? How much time did FDA spend at their place?" Colton asked.

"Just a day at Jacobson's. Same for Belvadere," he replied.

Jackie sat forward in his chair, put his elbows on the desk and turned a large paperclip over in his hands. Colton stepped into the office. and Jackie stood up and walked around to the front of his desk. The two stood face-to-face, silent until finally, he spoke.

"We're going to stay legit until I give the order to resume operations, got that?" he said.

"Got it." Jackie answered quickly.

"My orders, Jackie. You wait for my orders," Colton said.

"Yep," Jackie replied.

Colton studied him. Something about him gnawed at his gut today.

"Could be months, but we can't rush this thing. We have to make sure everything's blown over before we're up again," he said, looking past Jackie to the papers on his desk, searching for something, anything.

"Smart move, Colton. You handled this thing perfectly," Jackie said.

He was right. Colton had handled it perfectly, and now he would reward himself. The thought of Kristin eased part of his uneasy gut.

"I'm going out for a few hours, but I'll be back. Call me if anyone shows up," Colton said.

Jackie nodded.

"I mean call me *immediately* if any of those clowns show up here," he repeated.

"Absolutely," Jackie replied.

The ride through Valley Forge Park was pleasant and peaceful. Although the trees were mostly bare, the golden grass in the meadows rippled in the breeze, reminding Colton of the ocean sands of St. Bart's. He'd have to bring Kristin with him there some day. There were few cars in the parking lot when he got there. Colton pulled into a space and waited. He was excited but worried. This was not his kind of encounter and Kristin was going to have to work harder to make him feel comfortable. His phone rang as a red Mercedes convertible with a blonde drove past him and parked about ten spaces to his right.

"Wait until all the cars are gone. It's nicely deserted up the trail. I'll wait for you," she said.

He watched as she put the top up on the convertible, exited, and then headed up the trail and into the woods. Colton waited until someone drove off in the only other car in the lot, and then got out of his car and followed the trail.

At first he was aroused by her game, amused even, but the longer he walked, the more annoyed he became. The trail had become less defined, rockier, thicker with trees. He could hear the water rushing in the nearby stream, tripped over the pine needles and broken branches underfoot on the trail. Just as he was about to turn around and head back, he noticed a blanket laid out at the base of a large pine tree. A blue bag on the blanket leaned against the tree. He stopped and waited. Kristin stepped out from behind the tree dressed in nothing but a pair of bright red heels.

"I think this little wood nymph could use some company," she purred.

Colton approached and stood in front of her, waiting for her to do her job. She kissed him lightly on the mouth, then pushed on his shoulders and leaned him against the tree. She kissed him again, harder this time, shoved her tongue in his mouth, pulled her mouth away and slid her body down the length of his until she was on her knees at his feet.

"Close your eyes," she ordered.

He complied and leaned his head back against the tree. The musty outdoor smell relaxed him, prepared him for the pleasure to come. He felt her unzip his pants, and then stop.

"No peeking," she said sweetly.

He heard rustling, waited for her to pleasure him. Instead of her warm, wet mouth on his cock, he felt cold, hard steel against the bottom of his chin, then a deafening bang and excruciating pain. He didn't remember falling. He opened his eyes and saw up through the branches of the towering pine tree above, saw the remnants of leaves on the surrounding trees. Something oozed down the sides of his face, pooled at the back of his head. He heard gurgling. It was hard to breathe. Kristin stood over him, grimacing, laughing, pacing, and saying something.... He couldn't hear all the words.

"Not… smart…Colton … Never… cheat a working girl..."

He tried to get up, but couldn't move. He tried again. More liquid gushed down his face, his neck, and trickled down his throat. He could feel something soak into the back of his shirt.

"Help me," he thought he said.

She laughed.

"Help me," he thought he repeated.

She laughed harder.

He didn't feel his mouth move. He tried to touch his hand to his mouth. His hand didn't move. He closed his eyes. When he opened them again, she was still naked, leaning over him. The Palestinian appeared next to her. He couldn't tell whether he was really there.

"He is not dead yet," said the Palestinian.

"He will be soon," she replied.

"What did you use?" he asked.

"Mine. Yours was too heavy," she replied.

"Shoot him again. Use the same gun," he said.

"No. Wait for Jackie," she insisted.

The words jumbled up in Colton's brain. Could he hear them or was he making them up? He closed his eyes, opened them again. Kristin was dressed now, and the Palestinian was gone.

"Anything you want… Help me," he repeated.

She did not react to him, so he was not sure he had spoken. She leaned in close to his face, grimaced, and then stood back again. Jackie appeared next to her. Colton screamed and cursed him with every word he knew. He tried to get up and tried to pummel Jackie's with his fists. Jackie ignored him. Maybe he didn't hear him. Why couldn't he move? Why couldn't they hear him speak?

"Stupid cunt," Jackie mumbled and slapped Kristin.

"The fucking .45 was too heavy! I had to use my .22!" she yelled.

"You took his jaw out, probably lodged the bullet in his brain, but he's still alive," said Jackie.

"He will die soon," offered the Palestinian.

Colton tried to tell them to help him, tried to offer them money—more money than they would ever want. He tried to convince them to save him. No one heard.

Jackie and the Palestinian stood together. Kristin crouched down next to Colton. He closed his eyes. He heard voices, arguing, and a loud bang. Something heavy fell on him and crushed his chest. There was hair over his eyes, Kristin's blond hair. He smelled perfume. He gasped for air.

Jackie leaned in close to Colton's ear and spoke.

"I'm taking it all back, Colton," he hissed.

Jackie moved away and pressed something hard against the side of Colton's head. Colton closed his eyes.

***

Kat sat in the truck outside of Albe's until Bernie's whining got so loud she could no longer ignore it. All she could think about was Jimmy and how much she wanted to believe him. Why was he with Barnes in the first place? Though she didn't want to believe it, she couldn't shake the feeling that Jimmy was hanging around her just to get information to Barnes. When Bernie turned his whine into an eardrum splitting howl, she got him out of the truck and headed up the walk to Albe's frat house.

Martha was busy in the kitchen. Albe was whipping up drinks at the table. Kat took some time to clean up in the bathroom and change clothes before joining them.

"Don't you think you ought to help her?" Kat asked as she walked into the kitchen.

Albe made a sour face.

"No, Mrs. Vasquez. Trust me, Famosa women like to control their own kitchen. When it's Albe's night to cook, it's all his. But for now, it's all mine."

Kat glanced at Albe, who was vigorously nodding his head. She cracked a smile and counted her blessings. It had been a long time since someone cooked dinner for her, a long time since she felt like part of a family.

"I thought you'd be in a better mood. It's all over the news that you guys were at Barnes' condo today," he said.

"He's probably in custody now," Kat said casually.

Albe slapped his hands on the table and hollered, "Jesus, Mom, that's great!"

Kat tried not to gloat, but she did take a moment to bask in the glow of their praise. Jimmy still nagged at her. She still worried whether she would turn out to be the Mark Furman moment of the trial. She took a swig of her drink and grabbed a few chips and dunked them into Martha's homemade salsa.

"Yeah, well. Grabbing Barnes was only the first part. We have to flush out the supply while the manufacturers are gearing up to replace all the stock. Could take about a month…more depending on quarantines. Tough part is going to be making sure that patients with life threatening conditions continue to get their meds while supply gears back up. Unfortunately, I think we're still in for some tough days," she said.

"Not as tough as the Congressional hearings are going to be," offered Albe. He leaned back in his chair and tipped his glass to Kat.

"Yeah, well, Kneeley has already asked me to meet with him and some of the other Committee members to talk about what kinds of legislation needs to be put in place," she replied.

"Albe, you should be impressed! Your mother is a very big deal," called Martha from the stove.

"She's always been a big deal to me," Albe replied. He punched his mother lightly on the arm as she reached for more chips. Kat flashed him a look of mock anger and quickly turned away, to hide her real emotion.

"Whatever you're cooking smells fantastic, Martha," she said.

"Stuffed poblano peppers," Martha replied.

Kat's stomach growled. She savored the smell, took another sip of her drink and nibbled at more chips. Bernie appeared and sniffed around the table. Kat pushed him away with a sharp "no." Undeterred, he bounded over to Martha and she tossed him a couple of scraps. Now Bernie planted himself at Martha's feet waiting for more.

"You won't be here much longer?" Martha asked.

"Albe's not getting rid of me that fast. It's going to take another couple of weeks to wrap up the investigation, then I'll head back home," Kat replied.

"Good, then there's enough time for you to meet my family," Martha said.

Kat raised her eyebrows, peered at Albe and mouthed, "meet the family?" Albe tried to hold back a grin, but eventually gave up and shrugged.

"I would love to meet your family!" Kat said.

Martha finished the dish she was working on, popped it into the oven, and joined the two of them at the table. Bernie continued to stand in the kitchen and whine, until he finally gave up and sauntered out of the room. Albe poured Martha a fresh margarita from the pitcher and the three clinked glasses in a toast.

"Well Mom, your lectures finally paid off," said Albe.

Kat squinted at him and asked, "Which one?"

"You know, the one closest to your heart," said Albe.

Kat leaned back in her chair and looked from Albe to Martha and back again.

"I'm taking your advice and applying to pharmacy school," Martha finally said.

Kat yelled and shook her fists in the air, which attracted Bernie from the next room. She bounded around the table to hug Martha, but Bernie got there first.

"Imagine what she's going to be like when we get engaged," Albe said.

Kat stood still and looked at Albe, who pretended to ignore her.

"Albe!" Martha said, slapping Albe on the shoulder. "Don't do that to your mother. Kat, we've talked about it, but no plans for now. We've still got plenty of school left."

Kat smiled at Martha, then pulled Bernie off of her and dragged him back with her and made him sit.

"Couldn't resist, huh, Albe?" Kat scolded.

"You did pretty good with it, Mom," he answered.

Kat took another gulp from her drink and offered a little wink upward to Jorge. She knew her son well enough to know that Albe was sending a pointed message and she could feel her heart flutter a bit. This was her only child moving on with his life.

She knew it was her job to give her son wings; she just didn't want him using them to fly too far away. She consoled herself by remembering that they would be tied to Philadelphia for the next few years while they finished school and that she'd be tied here for a few more weeks wrapping up the investigation.

The timer beeped and Martha retrieved dinner from the oven and brought it to the table. Kat finished off her drink, but resisted another, concentrating instead on the succulent dinner Martha prepared.

Just as they finished, Albe's frat brothers returned and the noise level in the house escalated, helped in no small part by Bernie's barkhowl. Relaxed and stuffed, Kat realized she was too tired for all the commotion and bid farewell for the evening. She thanked Martha and gave her a big hug. She tried to say goodbye to Bernie, but he was busy with the frat boys so she just tugged lightly on his tail and waved to the boys. Albe walked her to the car.

"She's great," Kat said.

"I know. I liked her immediately," he replied.

"I can see why," she said.

"Yeah, she's a lot like you."

Kat smiled. For once she wasn't going to continue the questions, partially because she didn't want to know, and partially because she already did.

Albe gave her a big hug before bounding up the steps and back into the frat house. Kat watched until he closed the door. She sighed. There were so many feelings swirling around in her that she could hardly pin any of them down. Oddly enough, it felt like getting back to work would be a welcome relief.

She got in the truck and almost sat on her cell phone, which was wedged between the seat and the console.

On cue, it sprang to life, ringing and buzzing, and she scrambled to grab it before she pulled out onto the street. The caller ID said Tyrell.

"What's up?" she asked.

"Where the hell have you been? Everyone's been trying to get a hold of you for the past few hours." Tyrell was practically screaming.

"I'm here now, what's up?" she asked.

"You haven't seen the news?" he asked.

"Tyrell! Just tell me what's up!"

"Barnes is missing. OCI didn't find him at USA Distributors and either Jackie and the girl friend don't know where he is, or they're not telling," he said.

Kat resisted panic.

"Who's heading up the search?" she asked.

"OCI, but now they've got the FBI on the case," he said.

Barnes couldn't run for long. This thing he created has touched the entire country now and a good number of others around the world. Even with his connections, Barnes was bound to get caught. The question was, how soon?

"Where's DeAngelo?" she asked.

"They've got him in custody," he said.

"Kirk?" she asked.

"Him too," Tyrell replied.

Kat did her best to reassure him. After she hung up she slammed her hands on the steering wheel and yelled. She powered up the truck and took off to OCI headquarters and was halfway there by the time she finally got Thuyen on the phone.

"Sorry, I didn't have my cell on me, but I'm on my way over now," she said.

"Jackie's been released," he replied.

Kat held the phone out from her ear and stared at it, almost crashing the truck into a parked car.

"Ah, sorry. I thought you said you released Jackie," she said.

"Kat, I don't have a legal right to hold him. He's cooperating and so far, all of his information has panned out. We'll get back to him in the morning. Meantime, we've got all agencies looking for Barnes," he said.

"You're convinced DeAngelo doesn't know where Barnes is? You don't think these guys are working together?"

Kat could feel her heart thumping in her chest. She slowed her speed as she maneuvered the narrow Philadelphia streets with one hand.

"Kat, get some rest. There's nothing else we can do now. We'll get back at it tomorrow," he said.

Kat hated that answer. She always hated hearing that answer, even though she knew he was right. Still, it didn't sit right that Jackie was let go—not when Barnes was suddenly missing. It was too much of a coincidence and the whole thing was starting to smell like a set-up. Kat made it back to the hotel and headed straight to the war room. She stared at the papers scattered on the table, knew she would feel better if she organized them again, looking at every last detail. If DeAngelo was working with Barnes, she was going to find it.

For the next few hours she laid out chronology, chain of custody, warehouse connections, and timing, honing in on every detail. Her hand cramped as she dug the pen into the yellow legal pad to write long lists, circle turning points, and draw arrows connecting drug interactions and geography. Every detail triggered a memory of a report and the image of the face of someone whose critical medication failed them because of Colton Barnes. Kat tried to concentrate, tried to see just notes and numbers, but the faces crept up on her, piled up on the page. She rubbed her eyes, tried to clear them out and prayed that the demise of Colton Barnes would stop the steady parade of snapshots of dead people left in his wake.

Sometime in the middle of the night Lonny sauntered in, followed only minutes later by Tyrell. The three hardly spoke. Instead, they began to shuffle the papers around and lay out the case on the table in front of them with notes scrawled in Sharpie on papers from a yellow legal pad.

"Okay, what's confirmed?" she finally asked.

"Jackie said the manufacturing plant's in India," said Tyrell.

Kat scrawled "mfg India" on a piece of paper and ripped it off the pad. She placed it in the upper left side of the tabletop.

"Raw goods?" she asked.

"Could be Indian. Could be Chinese," said Lonny.

Kat wrote "Raw goods, India" on one paper, "Raw goods, China" on a second. Another rip and she laid the two new pieces above the first. Jackie had said that the goods were coming in by boat in containers, plastic wrapped in 55-gallon drums.

Kat wrote "container ship" on another piece of paper, ripped it and placed it below the manufacturing paper.

"All the equipment was in the warehouse?" she asked.

"Rolls of counterfeit labels and packaging came in by container too," said Tyrell.

"Perfect match to the manufacturers' too. These guys are good," added Lonny.

"Jesus!" Kat shouted. She shook her head in disgust and tossed the pad on the table. She could feel the anger rising, but she pushed it down, saving it for her face-to-face with Barnes.

"What's the range of goods?" she finally asked.

Lonny sat silently scratching notes on his own pad. Tyrell now inched away from Kat, chin on his chest, peering at her with raised eyebrows.

"What are they?!" she yelled, slapping her hand on the table.

Tyrell gestured to Lonny who puffed up his cheeks and exhaled before answering.

"It's easier to tell you what's not involved," said Lonny.

"Go on," she said.

"Erectile dysfunction, birth control, and some diabetes medications," finished Lonny.

Kat ran the words over and over in her head before finally speaking.

"Specialized baby formula too?" she asked.

"Listen, Kat, we got this guy. You can't get yourself all tied up—" Tyrell began.

"Baby formula, right?" she barked.

Lonny nodded.

"Pain meds, heart medications, anti-hypertensives, chemo, anti-rejection…" the words tumbled out, and as they did, the faces of the dead and dying marched across her brain, ending with Jorge. He was as real to her as Barnes' other victims. All over again, she smelled a whiff of his dying body, saw the sadness in his eyes, felt his cold, bony hand his hers, and heard his dying breath.

"These guys better fucking find him!" she said as she slammed her hands on the table.

"Listen, ah, maybe we should get some rest," Tyrell said.

Kat stayed still, staring at papers, memorizing Barnes' scheme, digging for a reason. What kind of evil was this guy made of? She picked up the Sharpie and wrote "warehouse – NJ" on a blank sheet of paper, tore the page from the pan and placed it on the table. She began to write on the next paper and the next until Lonny and Tyrell added papers of their own. By the time they were finished, the papers describing every facet of Colton Barnes' counterfeit enterprise covered the entire tabletop and spilled onto the floor.

The sun peeked through the window shade and Kat glanced at the clock. Lonny had lain down on the bed some time ago and Tyrell had fallen asleep on the couch across the room. Kat continued to study the papers. She wanted to commit every bit of Barnes' operation to memory. She looked forward to grilling him on every aspect, perfecting the case against him.

***

Jackie walked away from Colton's body feeling neither relief nor grief. Hamon had his instructions: clean the area, get rid of the bodies, get rid of the car, and call when it was done. Then, the monies would be transferred into an offshore account.

From the moment Colton took over USA Distributors, Jackie had plotted to take it back. He had suffered the humiliations, tolerated the insults, bit his lip and held his tongue. He had also worked behind Colton's back to build his own set of partners, patiently waiting for the right time to make his move. Now, it was done.

Jackie had realized the potential of the Palestinian the first time he had seen him in St. Bart's. It was because of the jewelry. He had seen how moved Colton had been by this simple gesture, how easily he was swayed by a stupid gift. Once Colton had left the room, Jackie and the others had laughed at him, imitated how he gushed over it, and howled at how he thought it made him important. Jackie had approached the Palestinian as he and the others came to help him load money into his car. Instead of helping, Reggie stuffed packets of money inside his clothes. Gus and Stewart joined in. The Palestinian did nothing to stop them; he just continued to try to get the box and the money into his small car. Jackie shoved the others out of the way, ordering them to leave the man alone. They left and Jackie helped him get the box into his car and the Palestinian expressed his gratitude. That's when Jackie asked him to tea. At a restaurant on the other side of the island, far from Colton's prying eyes, Jackie had pitched his proposal to the Palestinian.

"Mr. Hamon, I will offer you more money, a steady stream of income. And, you won't have to come to me and beg. Private bank account, regular payments, no records," he said.

"This is a very generous offer."

Hamon silently stared into his tea for a long time while Jackie waited patiently for him to speak.

For this, you will want me to do something," Hamon finally replied.

"Yes," said Jackie.

"Something that is worth a lot of money," he said.

"Yes," Jackie replied.

Hamon nodded his head and took a sip of tea. He stared on into the distance and mumbled to himself. He looked back at Jackie and spoke.

"This something is what?" he asked.

"Get rid of Colton Barnes," Jackie said flatly.

Jackie had left Hamon to work out the details himself, knowing that the less he knew, the safer it would be. An angry Kristin had showed up to muddle things up just as Hamon was closing in.

"She could be very useful," Hamon suggested as he and Jackie stood in the parking lot of an all-night diner in South Philadelphia. It was late. He had picked Hamon up from where Reggie dropped him earlier. "I was ready tonight. Only the fiancé was home at first."

"His flight was delayed," said Jackie.

The two men watched as a carload of teenagers tore into the parking lot in a sedan too small for their numbers. There was a burst of noise and commotion as the teenagers stumbled out of the car and moved through the parking lot to the front doors of the diner. The parking lot was silent again.

"She was very nice, the fiancé. He should have been more respectful of his woman," said Hamon.

"He should have been more respectful of a lot of people," Jackie mumbled.

Hamon shifted his stance. Jackie watched through the diner window as the gaggle of teenagers piled into a booth by the window. He thought back to the days when he and Colton and Langford sat in that same booth.

"Kristin will lure him to the park tomorrow," Jackie said.

"You trust that she will do this?" Hamon asked.

"No. I trust that you will make sure it gets done," Jackie replied.

Hamon slowly nodded. "He is your partner, yes? Your friend?" he asked.

Jackie turned his gaze from the teenagers in the diner to Hamon. The man, a self-described terrorist, was softer than Jackie anticipated. Maybe the deep lines on his face and his stooped posture explained that, but Jackie needed him to be a harder man.

"Business partner. Don't ask why," Jackie replied.

Hamon exhaled loudly. Jackie refused to look at him, instead turned back to the teenagers in the diner.

"To do evil in the name of goodness is forgiven. To do evil in the name of nothing is not," said Hamon.

Neither Hamon nor Jackie had counted on Kristin screwing up. Still, Jackie was glad to have had the chance to face Colton himself. Now, he walked down Mount Misery Trail to the parking lot past Colton's car to Kristin's. He popped the trunk, pulled a plastic bag out of his pocket and stuffed his latex gloves inside. He put on a new pair of leather gloves, stashed the bag in the trunk and took off. At the closest McDonald's, he changed clothes and bagged up the gloves, shoes and clothing he had been wearing. On the way back to the office, he pulled onto a side street that dead-ended into the Conrail tracks where an enclave of young rail bums congregated. He tossed the bag into an oil drum already half full with trash, lobbed in a match and watched the fire rise. The kids nearest to the fire watched him; others wandered aimlessly across the tracks in their drugged stupor. He approached the bums, dropped some packets of crystal meth, turned and left. As he walked back to the car, he could hear them scuffling over the gift. He drove to the King of Prussia mall, left Kristin's car in the parking garage, and then walked through the mall to the open lot where he had parked his car and drove back to work.

***

It took another two hours for all the investigators to make it to the parking lot of USA Distributors. Kat arrived first and was met by a crowd of protestors carrying signs with the counts of the sick and dying and pictures of victims, especially kids. Rubano must have made enough out of the story that it hit the nationals and brought out the hunters. Interwoven in the crowd were a number of reporters shouting questions and cameramen shoving lenses up against the windows of her truck. Two regular security guys tried to control the mob. She sincerely hoped she wouldn't have to call in local police to back them up. She inched her way through the throng and pulled into a parking space to wait, trying not to look at the faces of the protestors or those on the signs. She checked the rear view to make sure the rest of her guys got through the bodies okay. So far, security was able to hold back the crowd.

She sat in the truck and waited for Thuyen and his team. The longer she sat, the harder it became to block out the protestors who paced and chanted just the other side of the parking lot. She fiddled with the radio, rifled through her notes, and even called and talked to Lonny and Tyrell in their car, but none of it sheltered her from the horror stories. They seeped in through the car doors and penetrated her.

"Murderers! Greedy animals! I lost my whole family…" Kat hung her head and willed Thuyen to arrive soon.

Finally, three unmarked cars pulled up to the building entry. Kat ran to catch up with them just as they finished cementing the entry strategy. The shouts of the protestors grew louder, and turned into taunts, accusations. Kat wanted to get inside the building as fast as she could. Sirens screamed up the street and past the protestors, stopping just inside the lot just past the line where the protestors clustered. Two squad cars with two local officers each exited the cars and spread out in front of the protestors, keeping an eye on the crowd. Kat entered the building, stopped, and let out a long sigh.

***

Jackie DeAngelo sat at his desk and went on about his business. He was in the middle of a staff meeting when the OCI agents arrived and politely entered. He took one look at them, turned to the staff, stood up and made an announcement.

"As you know, we, like all manufacturers and distributors, are under investigation. We may be closed down for a couple of days as investigators do their job but I guarantee you that you jobs are secure and that USA Distributors will stay open."

He looked at the faces of the employees in front of him and for the first time he thought about the workers at USA Distributors and felt proud. His father had built the company and Jackie had grown up in the business. Many of the faces in front of him had been there as long as he could remember; some of them were surrogate parents to him. He suddenly felt a twinge of shame that he hadn't been strong enough to stop Colton sooner. He quickly dismissed it by concentrating on how he would convince investigators that Colton was the sole proprietor of his illegal enterprise and that everyone here, him included, were victims.

***

The team of investigators scrambled around Kat and went to work. They combed through every square inch of USA Distributors, searching, documenting and verifying every single item on the premises. They followed already prescribed procedure, along with the detailed list Kat had prepared. Kat walked the facility, watching investigators, eyeing almost every inch of the place, imagining Barnes' operation, still wondering about the why. She had just finished her third check with investigators around the facility when Paul showed up.

"You here to collect DeAngelo?" she asked.

"Change of plans," he said.

She watched him carefully, noting the taut jaw. For the first time today she felt the effects of no sleep. She braced herself for whatever was to come next.

"What's the new plan?" she asked.

Paul slowly pulled the sunglasses off of his face, rubbed his eyes, and then spoke simply.

"They found Barnes," he said.

Kat could tell by his tone, by his entire manner, that what would come next was not what she wanted to hear. She hung her head and rubbed the back of her neck and her shoulder blades, waiting for him to continue.

"Go on," she finally said.

"They found him in the Schuylkill River, inside his car. He was chained to a girl. Both took bullets to the head, but Barnes' jaw was blown off too. Police and FBI are on the case now," he said.

His words sounded distant, as if they stood at the opposite ends of tunnel. Kat turned them over in her head a few times, trying to make her brain absorb them. She looked at Paul, then off to the distance. She closed her eyes, hoping to find peace. Her heart thumped in her chest. She tried to slow it down. She should have been thrilled that Barnes was wiped off the face of the earth, but all she could think of was the angry faces outside and those of the dead thousands. And how she missed her chance to face down Colton Barnes and find out why.

Chapter 11

SIX MONTHS LATER

Jackie took a table on the far side of the diner and waited for his dad. This was one of the few places they could go without being bothered by sideways glances and deliberately tossed comments by those who recognized him from the news coverage of Colton's crimes. He hid behind his menu, contemplating whether to order scrapple and eggs, pancakes, or both.

"I found him, sweetie," Big Jackie said to the hostess. She smiled, dropped a menu on the table, then left. Big Jackie took a seat across from his son.

"You okay?" he asked.

"Trying to avoid any confrontations," Jackie replied. He slumped down in his seat and hunched over the table.

"You heard from Daddy?" Big Jackie asked.

Jackie shook his head. "Called a few times. Never heard back."

"I heard he's gone pretty heavy on the bottle," Big Jackie said.

"Yeah, well. Wouldn't hold my breath for that guy to win a father of the year award or anything," Jackie said with a snicker.

Jackie bit the inside of his lip and thought about how remote the chances were that his dad would be considered either as the waitress took their orders and menus. Jackie searched for a way to begin a conversation with his dad.

"So, what's up? Why'd you get me out here?" Big Jackie asked.

"Things are tough. I'm not sure how much longer we can keep going," Jackie said. He slurped his coffee and waited from his father to hand him some words of wisdom, something that would help him save the business he sacrificed so much for, but his father was silent. Jackie Jr. was hopeful that his father would have something to say soon.

While he waited, their food arrived. The two had ordered enough to feed a family of four and the waitress had trouble finding room for all the plates on the tiny table. Big Jackie dug into his food and ate as though it would run away if he didn't shovel it in fast. He ate instead of talking. Jackie was uncharacteristically disinterested in his food. He scanned the room, caught a couple at a booth near them , whispering and rolling their eyes in his direction. He wondered whether it was the sight of two fat men with plates and plates of food, or if they recognized him from the news.

In the days after Colton's body was found, Jackie had hung on every word of news coverage, relished all the lurid details, and delighted in the depictions of Colton as the poster boy for absolute evil. He also worried that his lies would be exposed and he might also be taken down. But the longer the story went on, the more the authorities seemed content to stop their investigation at Colton. The public was satisfied that the culprit was caught and it made for great newspaper and magazine stories, prime time specials and

Internet blog fodder. Jackie just wanted his business back to normal, and that was the only thing Colton's headlines couldn't deliver.

"You're not gonna eat?" Big Jackie asked.

Jackie stabbed a piece of scrapple with his fork, dipped it in his runny egg yolk and jammed it into his mouth. As he chewed, he watched his father. His napkin, tucked into his collar, was streaked with the remnants of his breakfast. His fork moved from the plate to his mouth with lightning speed and Jackie knew that he was on his own. Big Jackie was not going to save the day with any perfect words of wisdom. He had nothing to offer his son but another eating marathon. If he could just check out the New Jersey warehouse, if there would only be a pallet of cash there, his worries would be over. If not? That was a question he answered by swallowing a forkful of pancake dripping with butter and syrup.

After too many calories and too little conversation with his dad, Jackie headed back to the office. Every time he pulled into the parking lot, he took note of all the empty spaces and winced. The only way he could keep the business afloat was to let go of a quarter of the work force, and even then, he was struggling to make the monthly payroll. He hoped that Colton's case would be closed soon and that no charges against him or USA Distributors would be filed. Then the FDA might show up one more time and publicly clear him, ending this thing once and for all.

He had gotten tight with Rubano and in exchange for information, had cut a deal with him for an exclusive. He closed his office door and punched Rubano's phone number.

"What's the latest?" he asked.

"Hang on." He could hear him shuffling around in his office and the background noise of a news room. It got quiet before Rubano got back on the phone.

"Case closed. The initial coroner's ruling stands as murder-suicide. It'll headline tomorrow."

"Based on what?" Jackie forced his voice to sound concerned while sporting an ear-to-ear grin.

"Ballistics tests confirmed the bullets in Colton's body matched the ones in Kristin's, which matched the gun found inside the car. Apparently a lot of evidence was lost when the car was submerged in the river. Off the record, considering all the other evidence against Colton, I think the cops and the FBI kind of just figured good riddance, but you didn't hear that from me."

Jackie let out a long sigh. "It's over, huh?"

"Looks like," Rubano replied.

Jackie smiled and made himself comfortable on the leather sofa in Colton's old office.

"So, Jackie, thanks for the exclusive. Got me some big brownie points," Rubano added.

"Anybody talking anchor desk soon?" Jackie asked.

"Not at liberty to say," Rubano replied.

Jackie silently pumped his fist in the air; he had Rubano in his pocket and off his back.

"Let me know if you hear anything else, huh?" said Jackie.

"Sure, sure. Thanks again, man," Rubano replied.

Jackie hung up and relaxed into his seat. Hamon had delivered as promised. He'd used Colton's car to stage the scene and sold Kristin's to a chop shop. Linking the bodies together with a chain was some kind of special touch of Hamon's. Jackie wasn't sure what it meant, but he chuckled when he heard it. Bottom line was that the coroner made the call, it stuck, and the murder investigation was over.

The FDA was another case. Jackie had hired a gaggle of lawyers from Langford's firm to protect him and USA Distributors, just in case. But the FDA hadn't made any moves recently and now Jackie waited for an official report that declared Colton Barnes the lone perpetrator of the crimes. They had already seized the counterfeit supply and equipment at the dummy New Jersey facility Jackie had set up and worked with authorities in India to shut down the manufacturing plant there. Jackie chuckled when he thought about the poor guys in the Indian plant who had to take the hit for what Mr. Chen and his boys in China were doing.

Jackie's jubilation at the news of Colton's closed case was short lived. Like everyone else in the region, the business took a hit from a shut down and the bad publicity, but he had the added pressure of being associated with Colton Barnes. He needed some kind of confirmation from the FDA that he was cleared of all wrongdoing so he could begin the painstaking process of rebuilding his clients. He sat at his desk and pulled up a spreadsheet, studying the numbers. He chewed his fingernails as he did. The durable medical equipment column looked good, the medical supply column too, but the pharmaceuticals were a sea of red ink.

He itched to take a trip to New Jersey and see if there was any cash left from Colton's enterprise still in the warehouse, but he hadn't dared to chance it until now. Without some kind of cash infusion, Jackie wasn't going to be able to hold on to his enterprise at all. He was startled by his office phone ringing.

"There's a Jimmy Kirk on the line. You want to take the call?" asked Betsy.

Jackie paused, trying to place the name. He'd gotten a lot of calls from guys in the business, most of whom were looking for some kind of angle on Colton's story. He wasn't interested in making any new friends or listening to any garbage about how his now dead partner screwed up the business for everyone.

"Tell him I'm out," Jackie replied.

He went back to his spreadsheets and fantasized about a pallet of dollars in the New Jersey warehouse.

"Sorry, but this guy won't get off the phone. He says he was a partner of Mr. Barnes'," said Betsy.

Jackie wondered what this was up to. He wasn't interested in talking to him, but he figured he could get him off the phone faster than Betsy.

"Okay, I'll take the call. Thanks Betsy," he said. The line went silent as she connected him with the call.

Jackie didn't wait for Kirk to speak. "So you got me on the line. Who are you and what do you want?"

"Jimmy Kirk, and I'm the guy you want to talk to."

"Why's that?" Jackie asked sitting back in his chair.

"Because I'm the guy that Barnes promised to expand with. I figure I waited long enough, but now I'm coming calling," said Jimmy.

"Look, I don't know what angle you're playing here—"

"Barnes already let me in on the particulars, the cash flow side of the business shall we say," said Jimmy.

"I don't know what you're talking about," said Jackie. He sat forward in his chair and was about to hang up when the guy kept talking.

"Nice job with the misinformation, by the way. I particularly liked the touch with the paperwork. Dummied up, I assume. Even Rack was fooled for a second. He's okay now, though. He was wondering why he hadn't heard from you since Colton bought it, but he understands," said Jimmy.

Jackie stopped breathing for a moment. He ran over in his again what he heard, felt the sweat bead up on his lip. He waited for Kirk to say more, but he wasn't talking. He left the silence alone. He wasn't sure who this Kirk was, but he wasn't anyone Jackie wanted to risk talking to.

"Who are you?" Jackie asked in a horse whisper.

"Listen, I'm on your side, Jackie. I just want to meet and discuss a few things," said Jimmy.

"Why would I meet with you?" Jackie asked.

"Because I can imagine you need a cash infusion right about now and I know how to get you one," said Jimmy.

The guy sounded too cocky and Jackie was afraid this was some kind of sting. If Kirk was on the up and up, he might have the answer to Jackie's problems.

"I'll hear what you have to say, but no promises," Jackie finally said.

He agreed to the meeting to get rid of Kirk, then worried. Was his phone tapped? Was his office bugged? Was this guy who he said he was, or an operative of the FDA or maybe the FBI? Jackie dug through his drawers, pulled out his box of Fralinger's salt-water taffies and started chewing. Before he realized it, his jaw hurt, there was a pile of wrappers on his desk, and he was no closer to deciding whether he should meet with Jimmy Kirk or not.

***

Kat sat beside Dan at the congressional hearings and tried to keep her mouth shut while committee members grandstanded and spewed their ponderous nonsense. She had looked forward the hearings, eager for the chance to finally convince Congress that the FDA needed more funding and more authority to make sure the American public was protected. The global economy made for a new world, one in which regulation was going to have to play a bigger role. If the casualty rate from Barnes' enterprise hadn't convinced them already, Kat was sure that her testimony from the front lines would. Only an hour had passed when she realized that she was trapped in an exercise for the camera and not a genuine attempt to reform the department. She was disappointed with Kneeley; she had naively hoped for better. The last day of hearings had ended yesterday and Kat had spent the rest of the evening snuggled up with Bernie, watching Mr. Smith Goes to Washington and finishing off a bottle of Pinot Noir.

It was tough to get out of bed this morning. The wine and the four days of hearings had taken their toll. But Bernie danced the pee pee dance around the top of the bed and on top of Kat, which finally coaxed her out of the sack. While Bernie rid the yard of anything that moved, she got ready to face her workday. She knew the committee would issue a preliminary report today, with the formal report appearing next week. The preliminary report would no doubt be filled with searing criticism of the FDA and its handling of the Barnes' disaster. Kat was just sick of thinking about how Congress so often thoroughly missed the point.

As she got dressed, she ran a number of scenarios through her head, excuses by which she would be able to avoid work today and hide out instead. She knew it was just wishful thinking and that, as always, she would hit the office on time.

"Dan's already in his office reading it," Maryann announced as soon as Kat got through the office door.

"You seen it?" Kat asked.

"Just some excerpts. You can guess," Maryanne answered.

Kat glanced at Maryann's raised eyebrows and knew immediately what was in the report. She kept walking to her office, with Maryann keeping pace.

"Finger pointing, accusations of incompetence, no new authority, no new laws," Kat surmised. "That about sum it up?"

Maryann nodded. Kat shook her head and kept walking.

When she reached her office, Maryann went toward her own office as Kat plopped down in her desk chair. The three-inch thick report sat prominently on her desk, on top of case files. Kat got herself situated, sipped her coffee, and then opened the report. She skipped directly to the findings section, leaned back in her chair and began to read.

After four full days of hearings on the biggest disaster in the medication supply in the nation's history, the committee's recommendations consisted of countless pages of blame. Not one clear change in authority was granted, not a single penny more in funding to hire additional investigators was granted, and not one more tool was offered to help clamp down on the overseas manufacturers. Kat shook her head, tempted to throw the report in the trash and fire off a heated letter to the Honorable Senator Kneeley. Better yet, maybe she should write an op ed for the *Washington Post* that would grab some headlines of her own. Maybe the American public thought their drug supply was safe again, but there were more Colton Barnes' on the horizon. Thanks to guys like Rubano, every detail of Barnes' operation was published, a perfect template for other wannabes out there. What the bad guys knew, as well as everyone else except for the United States Congress, was that the system still didn't have the right safeguards to stop this kind of thing.

"You still did a great job, Kat," said Dan, leaning against her door.

Kat slammed the report shut and tossed it to the other side of her desk, then looked up at Dan.

"You and I both know there's another Barnes in the wings, probably moving supply in right now," Kat replied.

Dan heaved a long sigh and stepped into Kat's office. He picked up a picture from her desk and studied it.

"Is this Martha?" he asked.

Kat nodded. She had taken the perfect shot of Albe and Martha with Bernie before she left Philadelphia and added it to the only other picture on her desk, one of Albe and Jorge at the beach she had captured when Albe was only seven. Dan set the frame down gently on the desk at looked at Kat.

"My dad was a narcotics cop," Dan began. "He shut down some of the biggest operations coming in from Miami, and made some of the biggest busts in the history of the department. And, as soon as he did, another operation started up and took their place. He never let it stop him. I'm sure it bugged him plenty, but he never let it stop him. Still got up every morning and did his job. Every single morning. Sometimes that's all you can do," Dan finished.

Kat stared at Dan who started straightening some piles of papers that were scattered around her desk. She watched him fuss over her desk and waited before she spoke.

"You're full of shit, you know that?" she said.

Dan cracked a smile, pulled his hands away from the papers and looked at Kat. "Doesn't make me wrong, though."

Now it was Kat's turn to smile. She knew he was right, but for now she wanted to wallow in her anger. Dan turned to walk out, then stopped at the door.

"Listen, we got some new recruits being trained on a site today. I need you to go over there and set a good example," he said.

Kat rolled her head around and groaned. The last thing she wanted to do was handhold during an on-site.

"Can't Maryann or Doug do it?" she whined.

"Gotta make sure they learn from the best," Dan said over his shoulder as he stepped out of her office and headed down the hallway.

Kat groaned again, this time louder so she made sure Dan heard it out in the hallway. She checked the internal calendar for the location of the training on-site, checked her watch and headed out.

"Miss Vasquez?" a voice asked from behind her as she crossed the parking lot. She turned and recognized the Rubano and kept on walking.

"Jesus, don't you have any other news to report?" she asked.

He scurried ahead of her, turned and faced her, walking backward as he spoke.

"How about an exclusive from the investigator's point of view?" he asked.

"Can't do it," she answered quickly.

"C'mon. This was one of the worst disasters in American history. Don't you want to make sure it doesn't happen again?" he pressed.

Kat was tempted to slug the guy. Instead, she watched as he got closer to the tail end of a truck that was too long to fit properly into a parking space.

"Don't you think that's what I do every day? Me and all the other hundreds of agents who are out there bustin' our asses every day?" She asked.

She finished her line just before he slammed backward into the truck and fell forward. By the time he had scrambled to his feet, Kat was pulling out of the parking lot and on her way to train new recruits.

***

Jackie arranged to meet Jimmy at a Starbucks in Haverford, someplace where no one was likely to see them together. The press had only given up hounding Jackie after his exclusive interview with Rubano a couple of weeks ago, but Jackie was still cautious to make sure he wasn't followed whenever he went out. Jackie got there before Jimmy, took his coffee and in a back corner of the room, away from the window and away from any curious ears.

A tall guy with gray hair and gray eyes showed up and scanned the room. Jackie assumed it was Jimmy, but figured they guy should have to greet him first. He sipped at his drink and stared out the window. The guy came over to the table and leaned over.

"Jackie?" he asked.

Jackie nodded.

"Jimmy Kirk," he said as he stuck his hand out to shake.

Jackie gave him a limp handshake and went back to his coffee. Jimmy excused himself to get his own drink and disappeared into the next room. Jackie thought about leaving now that he got a look at Kirk, but decided to hang around and hear him out.

Jimmy came back to the table, set his paper cup down and sat on the chair next to Jackie. He leaned in and got right to the point.

"We can call it a merger or a buyout, whatever way PR thinks we can generate the best feeling from the public and the industry. But we gotta get rid of the USA Distributors name. We both know that," said Jimmy.

"You said you were a partner of his?" Jackie asked.

"Your buddy wanted to buy me out and get into the nursing home business. Figured it was easy pickings, not much scrutiny, you know?" Jimmy replied.

Jackie was still cautious around this guy, wasn't exactly sure that he could trust him. Either he was brilliant, or he was on a suicide mission and too stupid to know it. His research told him that Jimmy's company was facing their own financial problems, but so far Jimmy hadn't admitted to that.

"What's in it for you, Jimmy?" he asked.

"Oh, I think you know the answer to that, Jackie. Just a smart business move," Jimmy replied.

He sipped at his coffee while Jackie studied him. He watched out the window as the cars pulled in and out of the parking lot. He waited.

"Heard some word that you guys are in financial trouble. Wanna talk to me about that?" Jackie finally said.

Kirk fiddled with the lid of his cup. "It's no secret. We got hit like everyone else in your partner's little fiasco. But we're back on line and there were a few things we did in the interim that kept our cash flow going."

"Yeah? Like what?" Jackie asked.

Jimmy plopped his arms on the table and leaned forward. Jackie put down his cup as Jimmy pulled a pen from his pocket and wrote on a clean napkin. When he finished, he turned the napkin around and slid it toward Jackie.

Jackie studied Jimmy first before he looked at the napkin. He still wasn't sure of this guy or any guy that would have been doing business with Colton. Jackie took another sip of coffee, put his cup aside, and looked down at the napkin. It took some time for him to synthesize what was written, and when he did, he stifled the impulse to chew on his fingers. He eyed Jimmy, then hunched over his cup and slurped.

"We've got global reach, if you're worried. There are a lot of big markets out there, including some countries that don't even have an FDA, you know?" Jimmy said.

Jackie caught his drift. He wasn't sure whether Jimmy was bluffing or what he wrote on the napkin was true.

"How do your partners feel about this?" Jackie asked.

"They've been looking for a way to get out of the business," Jimmy replied.

"What do they know?" Jackie shot.

Jackie bored into him with his eyes, but Jimmy didn't flinch.

"That I'm offering them a great buyout. Nothing else. Guarantee it with my life," Jimmy said.

Jackie sat back in his chair and looked past Jimmy, out into the parking lot. He had covered up the real parts of the operation to protect himself and his business, but he never really let them go. He told himself that he hadn't really contemplated continuing them, but he never closed them. He ran the numbers over in his head and blinked to get rid of the sight of the red ink. He sighed then leaned on the table.

"Payout comes out of your end of the deal. Not mine," he said quietly.

Jimmy cocked his head but stayed silent. Jackie slurped his coffee.

"It's a solid proposal, Jackie. You know it."

Jackie picked at his now empty coffee cup and contemplated his next move.

Counterfeit Cure is a work of fiction. Names, characters, places, dialogue and incidents are the products of the author's imagination or are used fictitiously. Any resemblance to actual events, locales, or persons, living or dead, is entirely coincidental.

AUTHOR BIOGRAPHY

M. Roman Slavin spent many years working in businesses that service the pharmaceutical industry while continuing to study and write fiction. She has been published in various small literary journals and her radio play "Becoming: A Symphony of Choice" was broadcast on WXPN in Philadelphia. For many years she has written a blog: readseethink@wordpress.com, which she describes as covering "topics of mass discussion".

Counterfeit Cure is her first novel.

Made in United States
Troutdale, OR
11/03/2026

56847376R00176